CHICAGO PUBLIC LIBRARY
JEFFERY MANOR BRANCH
2401 E. 100th ST.
CHGO., IL   60617
(312) 747 - 6479

CHICAGO PUBLIC
R02004 82945

CANCER

AN INTEGRATIVE
APPROACH

D1057175

CHICAGO PUBLIC LIBRARY
JEFFERY MANOR BRANCH
2401 E. 100th ST.
CHGO., IL. 60617
(312) 747 - 6479

CANCER

AN INTEGRATIVE APPROACH

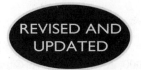
REVISED AND UPDATED

A Quick
Reference
Guide to
Combining
Conventional
and
Alternative
Treatment

JOHN A. CATANZARO, N.D.
Foreword by Dr. Joseph E. Pizzorno

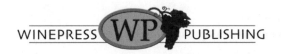
WINEPRESS WP PUBLISHING

© 2000, 2004 by John A. Catanzaro, N.D. All rights reserved.

Published by WinePress Publishing.
The views expressed or implied in this work do not necessarily reflect those of WinePress Publishing. The author is ultimately responsible for the design, content and editorial accuracy of this work.

No part of this publication may be reproduced, stored in a retrieval system or transmitted in any way by any means-electronic, mechanical, photocopy, recording or otherwise-without the prior permission of the copyright holder, except as provided by USA copyright law.

Unless otherwise noted, all scriptures are taken from the King James Version of the Bible.

Scripture references marked NIV are taken from the Holy Bible, New International Version, Copyright © 1973, 1978, 1984 by the International Bible Society. Used by permission of Zondervan Publishing House. The "NIV" and "New International Version" trademarks are registered in the United States Patent and Trademark Office by International Bible Society.

Scripture references marked NASB are taken from the New American Standard Bible, © 1960, 1963, 1968, 1971, 1972, 1973, 1975, 1977 by The Lockman Foundation. Used by permission.

ISBN 1-57921-499-1
Library of Congress Catalog Card Number: 2002116419

CHICAGO PUBLIC LIBRARY
JEFFERY MANOR BRANCH
2401 E. 100th ST.
CHGO., IL   60617
(312) 747 - 6479

R02004 82945

WARNING/DISCLAIMER

This material is published for the purpose of information and education. The information presented herein is in no way intended as a substitute for proper medical treatment and/or medical counseling. The author is not liable for the misconception or misuse of the information provided. This material is not intended to replace the services of a physician. It is not meant to diagnose and/or treat illness, disease, or other medical problems and should not be substituted for professional medical treatment. It is essential that you remain under the care of a physician.

Dedication

Dedicated to Anna, my companion in life, for her continued love, support, and stability, and to all my children for their love. And to all my friends who have prayed and cared—you know whom you are—blessings to you all! Special thanks again to Elizabeth Chapin, the co-author of the first edition.

May all those who read these pages find some help in their time of need, and may the ultimate objective be achieved—and that is the miracle of complete healing!

A Tribute

This book is also a tribute to all those who labor with compassion and empathy in the health care arena. There aren't any silver bullets that offer complete cure for all cancers, but those who put forth great dedication, have a strong faith in a Divine Creator, and genius, provide impetus toward a miraculous cure!

Also, to my patients who continue to fight against cancer, this book was written because of the inspiration you have brought to me as both physician and friend in your healing journey!

Table of Contents

Foreword

Cancer is the second leading cause of death in the United States. Prostate, breast, lung, and colon cancer occur most often and kill the most. And the incidence is increasing. And little progress has been made in survival rates when stage of diagnosis is considered. Clearly, the time has come for us as a nation and as individuals to start thinking fundamentally differently about the prevention and treatment of cancer.

Conventional cancer treatment by itself (with a few notable exceptions like blood and skin cancers) is not enough. Natural medicine by itself has not been proven effective in the treatment of cancer. However, together, substantially better outcomes can be expected. Conventional medicine has many effective ways to remove or kill cancer cells. However, the patient does not always survive the experience, and often the survivable therapy is not adequate to cure the cancer. And conventional treatment does virtually nothing to reverse the underlying causes that lead to cancer.

Into this grim picture comes the promise of natural medicine: herbs, nutrients, and lifestyle interventions, which help correct the underlying causes of cancer susceptibility, increase the vulnerability of cancer cells to chemotherapy, and help protect the immune system, liver, and healthy cells from the destructive conventional therapies.

Integrated medicine is not just about conventional medicine and natural medicine practitioners collaborating together; integrated medicine includes the full participation of the patient and honest commitment to validity and accountability. Ultimately, each of us is responsible for his or her own health; each of us is his or her best doctor. For this to occur, the patient must be informed and assertive. Equally important, every intervention and recommendation must be subjected to rigorous scientific evaluation. While hope and belief in wellness are critical to the healing process, wishful thinking does not help anyone.

In Spring 2002, the White House Commission on Complementary and Alternative Medicine Policy completed its two year study and submitted to the President and to Congress a blue print for integration of natural medicine into the health care system. While it is beyond the scope of this book to describe all twenty-one recommendations we made, of significant value here are the ten principles we derived to guide us in our visioning of an optimal health care system. These principles seem to be equally relevant to every person and practitioner committed to health and healing, regardless of disease, diagnosis, or school of medicine.

1. A wholeness orientation in health care delivery

    •   Health involves all aspects of life—mind, body, spirit, and environment—and high-quality health care must support care of the whole person.

2. Evidence of safety and efficacy

    •   The scientific method must be appropriately applied to identify safe and effective CAM services and products and to generate the evidence that will protect and promote the public health.

3. The healing capacity of the person

   • Each person has a remarkable capacity for recovery and self-healing, and a major focus of health care is to support and promote this capacity.

4. Respect for individuality

   • Every person is unique and has the right to health care that is appropriately responsive to him or her, respecting preferences and preserving dignity.

5. The right to choose treatment

   • Every person has the right to choose freely among safe and effective care or approaches, as well as among qualified practitioners who are accountable for their claims and actions and responsive to the person's needs.

6. An emphasis on health promotion and self-care

   • Good health care emphasizes self-care and early intervention for maintaining and promoting health.

7. Partnerships as essential for integrated health care

   • Good health care requires teamwork among patients, health care practitioners (conventional and CAM), and researchers committed to creating optimal healing environments and to respecting the diversity of all health care traditions.

8. Education as a fundamental health care service

   • Education about prevention, healthful lifestyles, and the power of self-healing should be made an integral part of the curricula of all health care professionals and should be made available to the public at all ages.

9. Dissemination of comprehensive and timely information

- The quality of health care can be enhanced by promoting efforts that thoroughly and thoughtfully examine the evidence on which CAM systems, practices, and products are based and by making this evidence widely, rapidly, and easily available.

10. Integral public involvement

- The input of informed consumers must be incorporated in setting priorities for health care, health care research, and in reaching policy decisions, including those related to CAM, within the public and private sectors.

Dr. Catanzaro's informative, authoritative, and carefully researched book is a perfect resource for those intending to, not only survive cancer, but thrive in their health.

—Joseph E. Pizzorno, ND
President Emeritus, Bastyr University
Co-Author *Textbook of Natural Medicine*

Preface

I am often asked what prompted me to write this book. I would say that the main reason for writing a reference work on cancer is to provide information that will assist one in making the most prudent decision possible. It is also essential that the information is updated, revised, and presented in easy-to-understand language.

I have written this work from the standpoint of what would I want to know if this one with cancer was a close friend or family member. I have also thought of what would I want to be counseled to do if I experienced cancer. I have treated many patients with cancer and have seen many transformations in their lives. It is a privilege to work along with those who have made it their goal to fight for the blessing of life. My patients have taught me that living in the moment is one of the highest life-lessons that is easy to know about but harder to practice. The practice of living in the moment comes when it is realized that there may be only a short amount of time remaining on this earth.

How Did It All Begin?

I am also often asked, "How did you start Health&Wellness Institute®, Inc.?" When I was a young child there were three things I wanted to be when I grew up: a doctor, an astronaut, and a baseball player.

As I watch my younger son play, he imitates the way ballplayers bat, run, and field. He has a natural talent. It reminds me of the days in the Bronx where I grew up playing baseball all year long in all kinds of weather. During the winter months, we lost so many baseballs in the snow that in the spring we would collect buckets of balls all over the place on the fields we had played on. Well, I got to play a lot of baseball during my childhood and teenage years.

Growing up, I remember watching just about every space mission on television. I had every part of the command and lunar module memorized. Every time I went to the public library I checked out books on space, flying, medicine, and baseball. I remember fantasizing about walking on the moon with the slow motion movements and sound effects. To this day it all still fascinates me.

There was one persistent thing, however, that never left me alone and that was becoming a doctor. It appeared to be impossible because of the great expense of the schooling involved. I had worked in the family business, starting at a young age. I spent countless hours with my grandfather going to the fish market in the Bronx, a family-owned business in operation for over seventy-five years. My family wanted me to stay in the business. I wanted to become a doctor. God had the same plan in mind for me that I did.

I completed my high school years while working in the family business. I went to work during the day and to school from 7:00 P.M. to 11:00 P.M., four days a week, until I completed and received my diploma. Little did I know that this was the beginning of my training program, initiated by God, to prepare me for my life's biggest challenge—completing medical school, a goal that seemed to grow more and more distant.

My early adult years were tumultuous, and I had many family issues. So I decided to get married to a girl (nineteen years old at the time I met her) while attending high school. At first glance I knew we were going to be together, sharing a lifetime together! Of course, during that time I don't believe we fully understood what we were doing. What did marriage mean? Well, I'll tell you we learned mighty quickly! As soon as we tied the knot, I went off to United States Air Force training, and we didn't see each other for several months.

I figured that if I couldn't fulfill the one dream of being a doctor I could at least begin to fulfill another by being around airplanes and maybe eventually going into space. Well, I had the best job in the Air Force—to keep those planes flying! I learned complex aircraft systems and worked for a recon wing. I served honorably and that ended my Air Force career. (When God has other plans for you, everything else becomes part of the training program.) I learned many things in the Air Force that even help me today. However, this was not the place for me, either.

We eventually moved to Seattle. We already had two children at that time, and I was struggling to find a job. I remember spending many hours with a friend (an assistant pastor) from church during that time. He also was trying to find extra work. Our church friends (the pastor and his wife) became very important to our lives, and they helped us in many ways. My pastor became a mentor for me and helped me learn to stay steady under pressure. My wife's father and mother were also helpful in many ways in establishing our clinic. My wife and I saw these things as God's hand on our lives, and she was the most prominent voice that God worked through to assure me that a new training program was on the horizon.

In the process, God called me to Christian ministry, and I began to prepare for this. I always knew intuitively that it was to be a healing ministry. I completed the program in five years and was ordained as a minister in the Church of the Nazarene.

One fine morning, my wife Anna came to me and said that God had been assuring her that He was going to bless me with my desire of becoming a doctor. My youngest daughter at the time, Angela, became ill with pneumonia and had serious bouts with asthma. We went to the emergency room on many occasions and nothing helped her. I searched for answers and became aware of a natural health clinic, namely Bastyr, and that they were doing natural treatments for asthma. We took her there, and within one month, my daughter was doing significantly better. This method of healing appealed to me because they listened to our concerns and spent time working on getting Angela well. I told Anna that this is the type of doctor I wanted to be. This began my journey.

I began to work on the required prerequisite science courses during the day and I worked for the Boeing Company at night. I worked and went to the community college for two years; my family saw me for less than an hour a day. Then I received a letter of acceptance from Bastyr University. I need to mention here that until I received this acceptance letter I pounded on the door of the academic dean's office many times! Dr. Ron Hobbs became my greatest friend, and to this day when he sees me he tells me, "I remember when you first came to my office with that grin on!" He said there was no way he was going to turn me away and deny me admittance to Bastyr. Thank you, God, for this man.

The university's president at the time, Dr. Joseph Pizzorno, welcomed me on board, and a new journey began. Dr. Pizzorno is a very effective communicator and mentor, and we have had several discussions on the importance of creating a new model in health care. To this day, I ask his counsel and advice on any new challenge that may come along that can change the course of health care.

My wife became very ill my second year into medical school and was not able to do the things she was able to do before an extreme fatigue came upon her. This is when I experienced what it meant to be compassionate and empathetic in ministering to someone who is ill. This someone, whom I love with all of my heart and soul, not being able to function was overwhelming at times. I became intimately familiar with what it meant to be a mother of five children and all that it required because the load was all on me. I wanted to be there for Anna and the children, and I did the best I could while working and completing the program. This is the place where I learned the deep soul and spiritual significance of healing!

Upon completing five years at Bastyr, I was faced with another huge challenge—starting a practice. This is something they didn't cover at Bastyr too well. Through my training experience, I worked with some pretty dynamic physicians who all encouraged me but who always said that the only way I could survive was by joining a large group practice.

But this was not going to work because these places didn't take in naturopathic physicians, and even currently there are limited numbers of groups that do this. The only option I had was to start my own practice. Well, the next logical place to go was to the bank and get some money, right? Wrong! The bank doesn't lend you money unless you prove to them you don't need it, and they want to know if you have any assets they can take just in case something goes sour. The bank was not an option.

One large medical group wanted to take me in, but I got a clear picture ahead of time what it would be like there. They wanted me to see thirty patients a day, and I was not even contracted with them yet. I knew that this was not the way to go. It would defeat the reason why I became a different type of physician.

I started my practice in my home (thanks to my wife and children for making this possible). I'll tell you, some of our greatest memories happened when the practice was in our home! While I was seeing patients, my kids would roller blade and ride bikes on the deck above. The dog would bark, the birds were always chirping. Patients wanted to know what was cooking for dinner. Many times patients would smell cookies baking and go upstairs after their visit was done, keeping Anna company, while she was baking.

Our waiting area wasn't very big so patients would stray to various parts of the house. We also had people showing up on our doorstep after 10 P.M., asking if they could pick up their medicines, not to mention how the phone would ring at all hours of the night. One person called at one in the morning to tell me they had stubbed their toe and wanted to know if they should go to the emergency room. I look back now and find it humorous, but at the time it wasn't.

We had one patient who had difficulty going to the bathroom, and I worked with her to help remedy this difficulty. Unfailing, my youngest daughter who was just potty trained would yell out for some one to assist her. She would yell for her sister, "I made poop!" To which my patient replied, "Oh, I wish I could do that right now!" My kids were part of my patient's healing on many occasions.

Now we have a beautiful clinic thanks to a significant contribution of my wife's father and mother. My amazing daughter, Jennifer, spent many years of training while Dad had the office in the home and by working for a doctor friend's office for a few years as office receptionist. Jenny is now our clinic manager.

When we first began our journey, we often had "duels," usually when we finished seeing patients—and oops!—a few times when patients were right outside the door! When Jenny first began working with me, I thought that she was to be at my disposal all the time. Well, she and her mom began to train me in an aspect I hadn't learned at Bastyr. No, I was not supposed to bother my daughter when she was in her room, which happened to be right next to my office, where I would see patients.

As a matter of fact, some patients (because of my example) would open the door to Jenny's room to see if she could answer their questions. After that happened one too many times, my daughter took me aside, and in a very commanding tone said, "That's it! This is not happening any more!" Can you just hear it? Wow! Did I learn quickly after that! My pastor used to tell us that if we could make it through the first three years without killing each other we would be all right! Thanks, Pastor, for those words of wisdom.

I tell you, we have entertained my father-in-law, as well as others, on many occasions with these stories. Tears and laughter come to me as I tell you this brief story of how we arrived where we are now. Thank you, Jenny, for helping me learn some valuable things. My wife assists in the day-to-day operations, Jennifer works as clinic manger, my other children, Angela and Adella, assist in administrative duties, and Vinny fills in where he can.

Now we have three other doctors besides me and six administrative staff all working together to achieve the goal of administering personalized health care, and we continue to move forward in achieving the great mission designed by God for the future of Health&Wellness Institute®.

I understand what it means to go through the trying times of life. All of us have some moment that we remember has tried every ounce of our life energy. If you haven't, then count your blessings and thank God for His tender care of you. But what counts in life is how you are remembered and what posterity you have left behind for the generations after you to embrace and carry forward. One of the highest privileges for me is to practice living in the moment with my wife, children, and friends. And I also count it a privilege to work with my patients who value the sacred blessing of life and fight to keep it. Of course, the rest is up to God!

God bless,
Dr. John

In Memory of the Doctor Who Dared to Be Different

Lois Berry wrote a book with this title that moved me to tears as I read. It is about a man who sacrificed much to provide the best care that in his patients' own words were "empathetic, compassionate, loving, encouraging, and hopeful." Dr. Glenn Warner, a remarkable oncologist, was different from his peers in the medical community because he did not accept the status quo. Hundreds of his patients have survived cancer, and many of his colleagues could have learned great prudence, empathy, and medical expertise, if they had been willing to learn from this man instead of minimizing his influence.

Dr. Warner was determined to the end of his life to battle against an unjust system of where healing becomes a crime. Dr. Warner was willing to use conventional and integrative treatment if it demonstrated hopeful results and honored the "first do no harm" of the Hippocratic Oath. Dr. Glenn Warner died on November 11, 2000, after a long oppressive battle with state government, legal personnel, and medical doctors who refused to hear the truth!

Dr. Warner's work will continue to be recognized, and it is the opinion of this author that all of those who participated in the unjust treatment must seek forgiveness and offer condolences to Mrs. Warner and family, former staff members of Dr. Warner, patients who suffered interrupted care, and all of those who saw the truth but were powerless to do anything about it! God bless the Warner family and friends. And, Dr. Warner, your memory will live on!

Warning about a Cure for All Cancer

There are reference works on bookshelves that claim all cancers can be cured. I think many of us would not be opposed to such a miracle. These miracles do happen, everyday. However, there is not a single cure for cancer at the present time. In addition, there is not a single cause of cancer but a multitude of causes. Be careful of a work that proclaims a single isolated cause of cancer and a single cure. Cancers are not just caused by parasites, and it is not as simple as getting rid of those parasites.

An individual can do much to discourage cancer in the body by following a rigid diet and a disciplined lifestyle, but this alone does not assure a complete cure. Individuals that have been given this type of false assurance have died! Maintain an open mind and search out facts. Don't fall for the fads of the day. Outline a strategic plan that includes diet, nutrition, bowel health and elimination, eradicating, if possible, agents that facilitate cancer activity, and enhancing overall body system health. These and more are all necessary in fighting against cancer.

Most importantly, don't ignore the soul and spirit aspects of cancer. These play a crucial role in the propagation and remission of cancer. I remember reading a quote from a well known celebrity: "It's not the things that kept me up at night that got me; it was worry itself, and now I suffer a seemingly uncontrollable process in my body. Oh, how I wish I could turn the clock back on those troubled nights."

Chapter 1

The Natural Approach

The doctor of the future is interested in creating an environment that will enhance the patient's health and well-being. The philosophy of natural medicine provides the motion and the substance sufficient to achieve it.

The natural approach provides information intended to educate and promote a better understanding of the options for treatment in cancer. Understanding the principles of natural medicine will facilitate a favorable outcome, regardless of the health condition. Below you will find a description of the guiding principles of natural healing. It is essential to consider a whole-person approach when treating any illness, especially cancer.

Natural medicine has a definite biblical origin because the system places emphasis on the healing of body, mind, and spirit and the use of the best of God's creation in the form of plants, wholesome foods, nature's bounty, and rest. Good health is the greatest investment in all of life. There is a strong relationship between "health and wholeness" with "obedience to God and humility." There is no substitute for clean living and a right relationship with God. In my opinion, these are the foundational elements required for good health.

THE HEALING POWER OF NATURE

During the early part of the century, medicine was largely giving a small amount of medicine or even a placebo and letting nature do the healing. A lot more emphasis was put on nature's ability to do the work of healing. We shouldn't underestimate the healing power of nature. Of course, God is the Creator of all nature and can utilize such a powerful force to work a miraculous work of healing. Personally, I have seen this power manifested on behalf of individuals that I have had the privilege of treating. Don't let medical science stand in the way of your hope of healing. Medical science focuses in on disease, prognosis, and survival rate and has a high emphasis on technology and its advancement. New development and hopeful therapies I'm in favor of but not at the expense of healing.

VIEW THE WHOLE PERSON

When considering the vitality of healing, there should be the realization that every individual is made up of three distinct parts:

- body—the part of us that has a physical being, or presence;

- soul—the part of us that contains the mind, volition, and emotions;

- spirit—the part of us that contains the essence of all life. The very breath of our being. A very mysterious part of ourselves. With no spirit, there is no life!

Balanced healing will involve all these parts of our existence. Often what is encountered is emphasis on the physical and/or the emotional alone, and all the rest is either ignored or neglected. If the mind is sick, the body is sick. If the spirit is broken, the mind and the body suffer right along. It is so vital to consider all parts of the person in order to facilitate healing.

IDENTIFY THE UNDERLYING CAUSE

Symptoms are a person's warning mechanism to tell us that something is out of balance or seriously impaired. Treating symptoms only may provide temporary relief from an underlying health condition, but the cause of the symptoms remains. It is essential to search for the underlying cause of a disease, rather than simply suppress the symptoms.

Though the emphasis of this book is on physical causes and treatment, many symptoms of ill health may also be caused by emotional or spiritual factors. I recommend you consult with a physician who is committed to discovering root causes of an illness on every level. This includes in body, in mind, and in spirit. Often, cause is neglected and symptoms become the focus of treatment. A patient came to my office with abdomen pain and yellowish/green-colored skin; she called her physician and he said it was probably kidney stones. He suggested a natural treatment alternative. I did comprehensive lab testing and it turned out to be pancreatic cancer. Identifying the cause requires investigation, and it is extremely dangerous when we do not listen to the individual suffering with the health problem and recommend a treatment that misses the mark entirely.

TAKE RESPONSIBILITY FOR YOUR HEALTH

The primary role of the physician is to teach and facilitate a person's health and well-being. The proper meaning of the Latin word for "doctor" means "teacher." It is not the doctor's responsibility to do the healing or make the changes necessary to facilitate healing. The very first and crucial step toward health and healing is taking responsibility. When it comes to individual health we must be put in the driver's seat. We need to make those decisions that will help transform our illness. Maybe this transformation is learning how to live in the moment and enjoy living. This is contrary to the experience we encounter in today's world. Taking responsibility is the first active step toward healing.

Health and Wellness

Health and wellness is a journey and a life-long pursuit. Whatever it takes to stay healthy should be our commitment. Health is the most valuable investment you will ever have. It is the greatest investment you can enjoy, and the principles of healthy living can be passed on from generation to generation. Yes, the greatest blessing of life is health and well-being, and there is no measurable material sum that can compete with it. There is a Bible saying: "The blessing of the Lord it maketh rich and He addeth no sorrow with it." (Proverbs 10:22). The blessing of health is greater than the blessing of wealth. Many times I hear the story of how earthly pursuits and careless living damage health, well-being, family unity, and the opportunity of living in the moment. Probably the best advice I can give here is to work hard not to let it happen! Pray earnestly for divine guidance to change the old patterns. Take action to change and become a person of faith. It is not fate that makes an individual well. Fate is at the root of what is fatal. It is faith that makes wellness possible!

WHY ILLNESS AND SUFFERING?

Illness can strike at any time and happen to anyone. Many good Christians have been affected by serious illness for reasons not easily explained or understood. Young and old alike are not spared from illness. However, there is a living and blessed eternal hope for the follower of Christ. There are various causes of sickness and disease, and when an individual begins to question, Why me, God?, God is obliged to answer in ever so gentle ways. There are a variety of reasons for illness, and this subject would require a complete separate work, which this author intends to write at a future time. However, briefly, I will describe some of these reasons for illness. In chapter fourteen, I talk about the healing journey and how one can find hope in the midst of suffering.

Wrong Choices and Careless Living

The Bible contains a word that many may have difficulty with, but it cuts right down to the core. The word *sin* describes all that offends God. In Genesis 2:15–17 one can read about the origins of sin and its consequence upon humanity. These consequences continue on in our current world, and they will not cease until the "new heaven" and "new earth," as the Bible makes clear, comes into existence. The Bible does plainly teach us that sickness can be the result of disobedience to God and such sickness is of supernatural origin.

In Deuteronomy 28:15–22, a clear picture is given by God of what to expect if disobedience and careless living remains:

> But it shall come to pass, if thou wilt not hearken unto the voice of the LORD thy God, to observe to do all his commandments and his statutes which I command thee this day; that all these curses shall come upon thee, and overtake thee: Cursed *shalt* thou *be* in the city, and cursed *shalt* thou *be* in the field. Cursed *shall be* thy basket and thy store. Cursed *shall be* the fruit of thy body, and the fruit of thy land, the increase of thy kine, and the flocks of thy sheep. Cursed *shalt* thou *be* when thou comest in, and cursed *shalt* thou *be* when thou goest out. The LORD shall send upon thee cursing, vexation, and rebuke, in all that thou settest thine hand unto for to do, until thou be destroyed, and until thou perish quickly; because of the wickedness of thy doings, whereby thou hast forsaken me. The LORD shall make the pestilence cleave unto thee, until he have consumed thee from off the land, whither thou goest to possess it. The LORD shall smite thee with a consumption, and with a fever, and with an inflammation, and with an extreme burning, and with the sword, and with blasting, and with mildew; and they shall pursue thee until thou perish.

After reading this I certainly wouldn't want to be on the wrong side of God, would you? God is a loving God, but He is also a righteous God, and He pronounces consequences toward any that offend Him! This doesn't mean that God causes illness to come every time an individual sins. It may take time for the cup to become full and God's patience abused. Remember it is God's desire for His creation to prosper and enjoy life, and all of these provisions have been made. He wants to bestow good things. However, He doesn't give good things for them to be trampled and carelessly handled. He provides a way out of the old patterns and habits. The requirements are conviction, repentance, confession, and the letting go of the burden of guilt to the One who can do something about them, and this is Jesus Christ, the Son of God, our Lord!

Familial Spirits

Often time I hear Christians say that illness is from the devil. Illness can have a demonic source, but not all illnesses paint a picture of demonic activity. Yes, all people, including Christians, can be affected by demonic influences, but the power of God is sufficient to destroy these forces of evil in an instant. The Bible does make a distinction between those that were afflicted with demons and those with physical illness. Not all illness is of demonic origin, though Satan can have a hey-day with any affliction, as in the case of Job! In 1 John 4:4, believers are given the assurance: "Ye are of God, little children, and have overcome them: because greater is he that is in you, than he that is in the world."

There are illnesses that are linked to ancestral influences. I like to call this the "spiritual genetics of illness." Countless times, individuals have said to me, "I don't want to experience the same ill health as my father or mother." The origins of this disease pattern can rest in many preceding generations, and the spiritual implications of such illness are very real. This doesn't mean that evil spirits are tormenting an individual. It is more that familial demonic forces remain hidden to keep an individual bound in fear or anxiety, which in turn can cause inner conflict. Webster defines familial as, "tending to occur in more members of a family than expected by chance alone."

The old saying here applies: "Familiarity breeds contempt, more so when it comes to handling things holy." Familiarity in spiritual matters can keep an individual blinded to the root causes of an illness.

Christians in general do not like to think about the possibility of this and would like to continue to believe that being a new creature in Christ Jesus eradicates all of that and there is no need to give it a second thought. Yes, we are new creatures in Christ, no doubt, but we still live in a fallen world where demonic forces exist. Adam and Eve in the Garden of Eden did not conjure up evil spirits. By choice they gave in! Afterward, they spent their lives fighting against forces of evil. The serpent was in the midst of the Garden, and he continues to reside on the planet, trying to confuse and confine us. As God brings deep matters of the spirit to light, we gain new power and freedom, and in turn the grip of the serpent is broken! This grip can be broken at once if God chooses to do such a work in a person of faith or it may be a process of time. Regardless, the awareness that the dark forces of the spirit world are complex and require the prudence and power of God's omnipotent presence to be broken is the only remedy!

THE DISPLAY OF GOD'S HEALING AND DELIVERANCE

There is always a special purpose that God has in an individual's suffering. Often time our disabilities and weaknesses are not viewed as opportunities by which God can magnify His glory. My friend in the faith, you are so special to God that even in your weaknesses and frailties God places His confidence in you! Phillip Keller in his writings (*What Makes Life Worth Living* ©1998 Kregel Publications) has said: "Too many of us have the wrong view of work with God. We look upon it as a grim bondage or a sort of serfdom. No, no, no! For when we truly come to know His touch upon our lives, and sense the sweetness of His Spirit at work in our souls, we are liberated into joyous experiences and adventurous undertakings." This miracle of healing that God works in you and through

43

you displays His power in your life. You should be asking, What is God doing through this experience? Instead of, Why is God doing this to me?

The apostle Paul was struck blind after he met Jesus on the Damascus road (Acts 9:8-9). Paul experienced the power of God in a new way. He saw Jesus and was blinded for a time. This was in part a consequence for his past sin, which forced him to face the truth. He experienced the healing from a Powerful Force that he was persecuting and discovered that this power was the reason he lived, moved, and existed. Can you fight against the powerful force of God? If you were to ask Paul this question, I believe he would tell you his life story, and when he was finished, if you didn't know the God Paul is talking about from the beginning of his discourse, there is no way you could resist the overtures that God is extending to you. It is the same force that Paul experienced on the road to Damascus, and with good sense you would give in to His overtures like the beloved apostle Paul.

The power of God was manifest in Paul's life in both the experiences of healing and deliverance and was heard about and seen across the land. Much amazement was experienced by the people of Paul's day, because he who once persecuted followers of Christ now became a follower himself. All of this demonstrates to the generations God's matchless power! He can do the same for you and through you—the world is watching!

Chapter 2

What is Integrative Medicine?

While nothing can substitute for the expertise of your own doctor,
no prescription is more valuable than knowledge.
— C. Everett Koop, former
Surgeon General

A harmonious relationship of the human body, soul, and spirit is
where healing begins. Healing is a journey that allows the "whole"
person to focus on wellness, rather than disease.

Integrative medicine is sometimes considered the same as alternative medicine. However, the term "integrative" specifically refers to the unifying of two healing systems. Both conventional (traditional) and alternative medicine (complementary) have much to offer in cancer treatment. Blending the best forms of both medical disciplines allows for a more comprehensive treatment approach. An integrative approach to treating cancer seeks to enhance the healing energies of the body and minimize negative reactions. Integrative therapy views the whole person and doesn't just isolate disease or symptoms of disease.

This book will discuss the options for integrative treatment of cancer in general terms. There are many types of cancer, and the best approach for the best outcome is in taking an integrative approach. In the treatment of cancer, it is essential not to focus upon the disease process or prognosis but rather focus on healing and facilitating recovery.

True integration also includes body, soul, and spirit healing. The whole person approach to healing does not neglect the emotional needs and spiritual well-being of the individual. This book includes these very important parts of healing. It is essential to focus on each of these distinct parts of human existence. God created us with body, soul, and spirit, and all are vital components of our earthly existence.

ALTERNATIVE MEDICINE

Mainstream medicine considers alternative medicine to be a system based upon empirical philosophy. In other words, many of the therapies do not have a solid scientific foundation, and how and why these therapies work are often times remains unexplainable. A slightly different system of validation is necessary to establish efficacy of alternative medicine. In most of Europe, the alternative medicine system is accepted, regardless of whether it can be scientifically proven.

As with conventional medicine, there are some questionable and risky practices that can potentially cause harm. Scientific validation doesn't assure safety. There were countless numbers of deaths from adverse reactions to drugs. Many deaths from negligence and incompetence are reported annually. Moreover, countless numbers of people are wounded or injured physically, emotionally, and spiritually from an indifferent and impersonal approach to medicine. Yes, mainstream medicine is guilty of all of this!

Generally speaking, alternative practitioners stress a holistic approach to health care. They often emphasize personalized medicine. They believe in treating the body, the mind, and the spirit— relying on noninvasive natural methods. This is a very beneficial part of this system.

For the Christian, the danger is in the various philosophies contained within the system of alternative medicine. Within this system of medicine, one may discover deep forms of Hinduism, Shamanism, New Age philosophy, Native American tradition, East Indian medicine, Traditional Chinese medicine, and more. It is essential that the Christian be alert and prayerful when attempting to utilize alternative medicine. The system of natural medicine, free from the foreign and alien philosophical views, is the closest form of Bible healing available today. It is necessary to cut the alien philosophy out and utilize the best part of the system. For example, the Chinese and East Indian herbs are some of the finest and most powerful in the world. We are not to throw out the entire content. We can extract by God's guidance and professional expertise the best part and throw out the potentially harmful. Finding a strong Christian physician that specializes in natural medicine is essential. However, there are very few of these specialists around.

When I was completing my medical education for naturopathy at Bastyr University, Christian believers were definitely a minority. I was in the process of being ordained and at the same time going through this medical program. God first directed me to develop the foundation to work with Christian believers from a faith standpoint. I learned very quickly under God's leadership what pitfalls to avoid! It was all part of God's masterful purpose to have me go through this process in order to serve from a point of expertise in matters of faith and medicine.

There are continuous efforts in progress to help validate the safety and efficacy of alternative medicine. However, all of these efforts may not substantiate the use of this system of medicine in its entirety for the Christian believer. What God forbids is considered harmful, and no amount of scientific validation will make it safe. The same rule applies for mainstream medicine.

We must remember as Christians that it is our obligation to care for our bodies and to be careful when choosing a practitioner in whom we place our trust. The Bible reminds us in 1 Corinthians 6:19–20: "What? know ye not that your body is the temple of the

Holy Ghost which is in you, which ye have of God, and ye are not your own? For ye are bought with a price: therefore glorify God in your body, and in your spirit, which are God's."

For the Christian, evaluation of the alternatives should be accomplished prayerfully and with keen discernment. Earnestly seeking God on the matter will bring clarity. God can lead you to the right sources and people that can give you the best information. This information will be factual, giving both the benefits and potential risks, and then you must weigh the evidence carefully. The decision to utilize or discard certain alternative therapies should always be one of peace in your own heart and with your Creator!

CONVENTIONAL MEDICINE

Conventional medicine, also known as mainstream medicine (Western medicine), developed in the early days from doctors making house calls, utilizing more natural medicine as well as folk remedies to cure disease. Over time sophistication and resources has made conventional medicine a very valuable system. However, by this same amazing progress, mainstream medicine has become scary at times. Medicine has come a long way from the Dr. Benjamin Rush and Louis Pasteur era. I don't believe it necessary to return to the primitive practices of medicine. We must acknowledge that diseases that have claimed the lives of countless people fifty years ago are curable today. This is the amazing progress of mainstream medicine, and we should utilize the best of it!

In order to better understand mainstream medicine, one has to honestly and openly evaluate the history. In many ways the development of conventional medicine has many sad stories, irreparable mistakes, and bad judgments as well as successes and scientific discoveries. Alternative medicine can learn from the past failures of conventional medicine and develop a strategic plan of validation to minimize potential harm.

Conventional medicine also has limitations. Care must be taken to preserve the rights and confidentiality of the patient. With increased genetic advancement, there is also increased risk of violating personal rights. In addition, there is increased risk of early termination of life due to genetic abnormalities. Another possible threat is an uncontrollable avalanche of genetic mistakes that can harm future generations. The Hippocratic Oath's first proclamation is "First do no harm." Yes, there is the potential for harm and limitations in Western medicine. There remain diseases like cancer and heart disease that continue to remain incurable. Both conventional and alternative medicine has much to offer; integrating the best of both systems is what is needed to produce the best possible outcome. However, it must be remembered that none of these systems are God. The Great Physician works the healing, and He will use the means that is consistent with His nature—and that is holy!

How to Choose Your Health Care Team

One of the most challenging aspects of your total care you may encounter is a health care team that works in unison to achieve the best outcome. Often there is a huge chasm between conventional and non-conventional providers. Both sets of providers must advocate for you and work as a team. Otherwise, your treatment experience becomes a continuous anxiety producer. Your physicians should converse together and keep communication flowing freely. There are valuable checks and balances in this, and it will assure that your team players are on the same playing field. Your conventional and complementary providers may include:

Conventional Medical Providers

Conventional physicians utilize western-based medicine, emphasizing chemotherapeutics, radiation therapy, conventional drugs, and surgery.

- Endocrinologist—specializes in the hormonal system and may be involved in initial diagnosis.

- Gastroenterologist—specializes in disorders of the bowel and is involved in the screening and diagnosis of cancers that involve the bowel.

- Internist—similar to a primary care physician, specializing in internal medicine.

- Oncologist/hematologist—specializes in cancer and blood disorders.

- Primary care physician—often the gatekeeper and plays a crucial role in monitoring your care.

- Radiation oncologist—specializes in the use of radiation therapy and will work with your primary oncologist.

- Surgeon—works along with an oncologist in excising tumors and can repair damage caused by cancerous lesions.

- Urologist—specializes in the genitourinary system and may be involved in initial diagnosis. Some urologists are also surgeons and may perform specialized procedures such as BCG and seed implants, in conjunction with radiation oncologists.

Alternative/Complementary Medical Providers

Alternative care providers utilize both Western and Eastern-based medicine, offering a wider variety of options. This can include the use of herbs (Western tradition, Chinese tradition, and Ayeurvedic tradition), acupuncture, nutrition, postural manipulation, homeopathy, massage therapy, IV nutritional, and chelation therapies, etc. A great benefit is that a complementary provider can be an advocate in your total health care, helping you to stay away from therapies that may be potentially harmful.

- Acupuncturists—practice Oriental medicine, utilizing needles to free meridians that are blocked. Good for pain management.

- Alternative medical physicians—medical doctors that have a specialized focus in alternative therapies.

- Alternative osteopathic physicians—osteopathic doctors that have a specialized focus in alternative therapies.

- Chiropractors—specialize in postural manipulation. Some perform reflexology in conjunction with nutrition therapy.

- Homeopaths—specialize in utilizing homeopathy, these practitioners can be osteopathic physicians, medical physicians, or naturopathic physicians.

- Massage therapists—provide massage therapy, which may include lymphatic drainage massage.

- Naturopathic physicians—specialize in natural integrative therapies, postural therapies, homeopathy, and nutritional therapy. There are licensed and non-licensed naturopaths. Beware of non-state-licensed practitioners.

- Nurse practitioner—a nurse that can perform primary care medicine independently and can have a special focus in cancer.

- Nurses—traditional RNs that work along with other providers in facilitating total health care. Some nurses specialize in alternative nursing and utilize non-traditional therapies.

- Nutritionists—specialize in nutrition and provide expertise in utilizing diet to facilitate health and healing.

- Oriental medical physicians—specialize in traditional Chinese medicine, which may include acupuncture and eastern herbal tradition.

- Physician's assistant—provides the service of a primary care physician and may specialize in surgical medicine.

All of these providers should

- demonstrate superior communication skills;

- demonstrate skill and experience with your diagnosis;

- work with you in achieving your goals in treatment;

- work with non-conventional providers to integrate alternative therapies that are most appropriate for your cancer;

- have information and resources on the latest research available in your case;

- blend their expert skills with a compassionate-based approach. This puts the soul back into medicine.

Your providers should view you—the whole person—and work together with you to address physical, soul, and spirit needs. Compassion blended with expertise should be the standard. After all, the service of medicine must minister to the physical, soul, and spirit. My best advice is to look for a provider that has this most essential blend of expertise and compassion. This in itself will be both healing and hopeful. Keep all of your options open and be sure that you check details that are important to you. For instance: Where the physician practices, what hospital privileges in case you need to be hospitalized, how they handle emergencies, how accessible is the provider and staff, what insurance coverage, etc.

Chapter 3

Can I Use Alternative Therapy without Conventional Treatment?

The best approach is the integrated approach: Blending the best that both worlds of alternative and conventional treatment have to offer.

Putting the soul back into medicine can provide hope, inspire life, and facilitate healing. It may be the vital ingredient needed for a miraculous cure.

I have many patients who ask this question: Can I use alternative therapy (natural methods) alone to fight my cancer? There are no simple answers to this question. I am not in the capacity to tell my patients that they should *not* use conventional therapies to treat their cancer. Any physician who is put in this position is in for trouble. My role as a physician is to educate and instruct and give my patients the tools that they need to make the best informed health care choice possible. Knowledge is truly power in the sense that it dispels ignorance. Explaining risks and benefits of a given therapy, whether conventional or alternative, is essential. Are cancers healed using natural methods? The answer to this question is yes and no. There are many cancers that have remitted using alternative methods and many that have not. The same can be said of conventional medicine.

In my opinion, the best strategy in cancer treatment is the integrated approach—combining the best that both worlds have to offer. That's an easy statement to make in general terms because the challenge begins when you begin to search out the best therapy for your particular cancer. It takes work and the assistance of trusted experts, family members, and friends. You don't fight this battle alone.

The best results in therapy depend upon many factors:

- type of cancer

- therapies being used

- diet and nutritional health

- discipline and tolerance

- emotional and spiritual health

- inner heart sense of what to do

- blending conventional and alternative care

Type of Cancer

There are many forms of cancer, and they all have different patterns and origins. There are also many books on finding the cure for cancer. Some of these can be very misleading and offer false hope, while others are very helpful. Cancer is a complex phenomenon that requires a comprehensive understanding. You must realize that there are no "silver bullets" when it comes to treating cancer and that there are many aspects of cancer we do not understand. In other words, it is not as simple as finding the single cure. Cancer, in plain language, is a word used to describe disorder and the invasion of boundaries, thereby adversely affecting the health of the whole person. It is extremely risky in claiming to have the "cure all" for cancer. Any health and healing practitioner who claims such would be able to heal the world and assure immortality, and we know that doesn't exist, as much as we hope and pray for the one cure to fit all.

What is the best way to approach this complex disease? The answer is four-part:

1. *Minimize potential harm and maximize healing benefits.* The therapies you choose to implement should enhance the body's ability to heal and reduce the potentially harmful effects. It may be necessary at times to use a therapy that has some strong negative effects initially but is highly effective against the cancer. The key is that the therapy should not be implemented at the expense of the individual. For example, chemotherapy, radiation, and/or surgery should be carefully administered, keeping in mind the health status of the individual receiving it. In my opinion, these conventional forms of treatment should never be administered without supportive therapy that addresses nutrition, immune health, and metabolic health.

2. *Utilize the least invasive means as possible.* Again, the most invasive form of therapy should be used as the last recourse if all else fails. The key is to do your homework and search out your therapy. Don't leave that choice with your doctor. Yes, you must draw from expert advice. But the ultimate decision is yours.

3. *Consider the whole (body, soul, and spirit).* Remember that your well-being depends upon a complex interaction between body, soul, and spirit. This trichotomy (three distinct parts) is what makes you the unique person you are, and it cannot be separated out. It is not as simple as healing the body alone. The medicine you choose should be medicine that ministers to the body, the soul, and the spirit. Cancer affects the whole person, and the therapy you choose should also.

4. *Rebuild, restore, and revitalize.* These three words are powerful. They all require input. In your journey of healing,

there are therapies that take away life. For example, when chemotherapy and/or radiation is administered, the aim is to kill the cancer cell that threatens the boundary of healthy cells, tissues, and organs. That is the nature of the therapy, and it may be the only thing effective against the cancer. However, this is a therapy that takes away life, and there must be a counter therapy that gives life. Rebuilding what has been taken away is essential when it comes to extending life. Restoration is necessary to renew life energy that is required to fight the cancer. There are various ways of doing this. Nature is an excellent way of restoring life energy. Positive prayer is an excellent way of restoring the life energy of the soul and spirit. If you are too exhausted, have a trusted family member or friend pray with you and for you. Revitalize your existence! You may have to learn to forgive and let go. You may discover that worrying never changes anything and that it doesn't pay to keep this as a pattern in your life. There are certain life issues you must transform and develop into new healthy coping patterns that do not adversely affect your total well-being.

THERAPIES BEING USED

Alternative therapy doesn't always equate to being safe. There are many potentially harmful therapies in the alternative realm. I had a patient who came to see me for a chronic cough that she remembers developing after a specific therapy. This therapy is considered to be an alternative to combating allergies and restoring physical strength. She received a series of peroxide intravenous drips. Afterwards, she developed extreme shortness of breath and a cough. Recently, she had a treadmill test to determine the strength of her heart. She had extreme fatigue because her lungs were not responding the way they should. I believe that the peroxide therapy had adversely affected her and damaged a portion of her lung. Whether conventional or alternative, great care must be taken to explore the type of therapy, the results it demonstrates, and the benefits and risks of the therapy. The ultimate aim of any therapy should be to increase the chances of survival with the best quality of life possible.

DIETARY AND NUTRITIONAL HEALTH

Diet and nutrition are the keys to good health. What you ingest is important. What nutrients your body is getting on a daily basis will certainly help beat the odds of cancer. With cancer, you may want to consider a "whole foods approach." This type of diet has fresh vegetables, cold water fish, and colorful pigment foods to restore health. Keep in mind that colorful, healthy foods promote healing. Juicing both veggies and fruits that are fresh and organic is something you should consider.

If you really want to fight the cancer, a macrobiotic approach that is very strict and requires much discipline may be beneficial. I have heard of many cancer cases that have remitted using the macrobiotic approach. Whatever you do, diet and nutrition are paramount in your fight against cancer. Some anti-cancer diet programs may not be compatible with your tolerance and personality type. In other words, some are able to follow a strict Gerson or macrobiotic plan and others would become overwhelmed.

Your food should be part of your therapy, not part of your stress. Making prudent dietary choices alone will greatly improve your healing. So don't go on a guilt trip if you can't seem to follow a certain plan that has been recommended. It is easy to recommend a plan; it's another thing to have to strictly adhere to it. On the other hand, don't use your lack of discipline as an excuse not to pursue better nutrition.

DISCIPLINE AND TOLERANCE

When experiencing cancer, you will find that you must apply a whole new set of rules to live by. Discipline and tolerance are two essential factors that are required for the best outcome. When you are feeling sick and worn out from the whole process, and you're tired of being the experiment for the advancement of medical science, it's hard to think of discipline and tolerance. I encourage you to stick with what you know is working and don't give up. Continue to thirst for knowledge, and implement the positive and let the negative go. If you are tired, maybe you just need to rest from the chemotherapy or radiation. Maybe you need to give yourself a break from all those vitamins and rest. Whatever the case, try to maintain discipline and tolerance, even with some timeouts. It's best for you and your health.

EMOTIONAL AND SPIRITUAL HEALTH

The Bible tells us that "a merry heart maketh a cheerful countenance; but by sorrow of the heart the spirit is broken" (Proverbs 15:13). Transform your thinking into terms of expenditure of life energy. More particularly, think of it in terms of soul energy and spirit energy. How do you want to spend your life energy? Realize that there are all types of "energy robbers" popping their ugly heads up to whittle away your most precious gift—*life*.

How do you preserve this life energy? The Bible answers this well: "Keep thy heart with all diligence; for out of it *are* the issues of life." (Proverbs 4:23)

What are the issues of life? There are many and they are varied, unique to each individual. But whatever they are and however you face them, learn to let go of those things that steal your life energy away. Transform your soul and spirit and renew your desire for living. A good bit of advice is to seek God, who knows all things and who made a perfect being fashioned in His image. Turn to prayer and give your anxieties and fears to the One who can do something about them. Let it go, let it go, let it go!

INNER HEART SENSE OF WHAT TO DO

Go with what your heart tells you. Don't ignore it. I had a patient who decided to treat her cancer just using alternative therapy.

She used it for months, and her cancer was progressing and taking her life. She came to me in much frustration and very ill. She was afraid to do any other form of treatment because of the horror stories she had heard. She also had friends who succumbed to the ill effects of treatment. I felt in my heart that if this dear lady didn't do something other than what she was doing, she was going to die. She was not ready to give up on life. She wanted life. I told her that she needed to act on her desire to live. I advised that she consider a mild chemotherapy regimen that has worked very well for her type of cancer. This woman is still alive, and almost an entire year has passed. She is much healthier than she was and recently came into the office very happy about being alive. We are still working together to help fight off the cancer, but this cancer patient has a new hope for living.

In another case, there was a four-year-old girl with whom I had the opportunity to consult. Her parents wanted to know the best approach for their child's cancer. They had been to conventional practitioners and alternative practitioners alike. They received some strange advice and implemented several alternatives. They wanted to know from me if I felt that alternative therapy alone in their daughter's case would be enough. I felt in my heart that if some other intervention was not implemented, their child wouldn't have long to live. The parents were fearful of what was to come.

I didn't offer this counsel because I didn't believe in the medicine I practiced. I knew in my heart this child needed specific health treatment. I suggested the parents consider bone marrow transplantation. As it turned out, there were two years of constant hospital stays and visits. There was the requirement of having a suitable donor, but there was no one in the family who was suitable. They had to use the bone marrow registry, which created an alliance for life with a wonderful woman who continues to be involved with their family. This beautiful child is alive today. Truly, this is a miracle of God that depended on prayerful counsel. Just remember to get all the required facts, then *go with what your heart tells you!*

BLENDING CONVENTIONAL AND ALTERNATIVE CARE

When considering an integrative approach to cancer therapy, it is important that you be informed about the treatment options offered in both realms. In order to have an effective treatment plan, you must have the following information:

- all of your diagnostic work up from all physicians

- knowledge of your current and previous conventional cancer treatments

- personal and family history

- what your goals and objectives are surrounding the treatment

Often times I encounter patients that do not know all there is to know about their cancer diagnosis. It is vitally important to know your history and the current details that surround your diagnosis and treatment. Such information will be crucial in designing an effective therapeutic regimen.

What important information must be known?

- the type of cancer you were diagnosed with

- the staging of the cancer

- the treatments recommended

- the possible beneficial or negative effects of the treatment

There is a system of tumor staging known as the TNM system. This system has the following meaning: T= primary tumor, N= nodes involved, and M= metastases (spread of the tumor from its primary origin). Staging of cancer is crucial when considering a treatment regimen.

I would recommend that you keep a specific journal on the details of your personal and family history and diagnostic information, including labs, imaging, and physician's evaluation. In this journal, you should also include your personal reflections of your journey. This journal will become a most valuable work that reflects details of your journey and that should be shared with close family and friends who love you and who participate in your total care.

There are many cancer types, and each of them has characteristics and affinity for certain body areas and systems. Briefly, we will discuss some of these cancers. I would like to mention here that the best approach to cancer treatment is an integrative approach. You probably remember me mentioning this many times in previous chapters, and I will continue to remind you of this, because while we discuss the cancers individually, it would be easy to concentrate on the disease process rather than the healing that must take place within.

Chapter 4

What Is Cancer?

Cancer has become so prevalent in our world that the term is often used as a word picture to describe anything that is uncontrolled, abnormal, and life threatening in our society.

Cancer is the second leading cause of death in the United States. Cancer risk increases with age, and it is estimated that two-thirds of all cases occur in people over age sixty-five.

Some quick facts about cancer:

1. cancer is an invasive, uncontrolled replication of cells in the body;

2. lifestyle and environmental factors are indicated as being the cause of about 60% of existing cases of cancer;

3. cancer risk is high in individuals who have family members with cancer;

most cancers require several years to develop; if the cancer is detected early and properly treated, most cancer patients have a favorable outcome. But, since cancer can be deadly, prevention should become a way of life.

WHAT CAUSES CANCER?

Currently, it is thought that cancer is caused by multiple factors. Many physicians agree that cancer has multiple interacting cancer causes. This is contrary to the scientific view of identifying single precipitating factors—such as genes or infectious organisms. Practitioners of integrative medicine know there is no single cause for cancer, nor is there a single cure. Cancer is caused by a gradual toxic systemic exposure and weakening of body systems (i.e. immune system). However, there are contributing factors that will be reviewed briefly and are listed below.

- chronic stress
- diet and nutritional deficiencies
- environmental toxins
- excess exposure to sunlight
- food additives
- free radicals
- genetic predisposition
- heavy metal toxicity (mercury, arsenic, lead, etc.)
- hormonal dysfunction
- immune-suppressive drugs
- intestinal toxicity and digestive imbalance
- oncogenes (genes responsible for initiating cancer)
- pesticides and herbicides
- polluted water
- tobacco and smoking
- viruses

Chronic Stress

Stress can be defined as a reaction that can potentially upset the function of normal physical and emotional health. There are various causes of stress, such as illness, pain, loss, grief, financial pressures, and so on. Chronic stress directly affects the immune system in a negative way. Stress is part of life and a continual health challenge. The stress load continues to grow with each passing decade. Many Americans today experience stress from the overwhelming job pressures in a fast-paced corporate culture. Under emotional distress, the brain releases many signals to produce certain hormones that can weaken the immune response. Cancer activity can be accelerated in the presence of these chemicals. Research confirms that emotional stress can increase your susceptibility to illness. Chronic stress that is unrelieved can begin to weaken body systems and suppress vital function.

Diet and Nutritional Deficiencies

The types of foods we eat profoundly influence our health. According to the National Academy of Sciences, 60% of all cancers in women and 40% of all cancers in men may be caused by dietary deficiencies and nutritional factors.[1] Some of the negative factors in diet are listed below.

- excessive intake of meat products
- excessive intake of processed and smoked foods
- decreased vegetable and leafy green intake
- contaminated fish and seafood intake
- excessive fat intake
- excessive sugar intake
- excessive alcohol and caffeine consumption
- inadequate hydration (not drinking enough water)

- inadequate essential fatty acid intake (omega 3, 6, and 9)

Nutritional imbalances may increase cancer risk and facilitate degenerative disease. A wholesome diet with healthy foods is the foundation of good health.

Environmental Toxins

There is a continuous challenge to keep environmental pollutants under control. The Environmental Protection Agency (EPA) estimates that as many as ten thousand cancers a year in the United States can be attributed to indoor air pollution. The EPA cannot begin to calculate how many cancer cases are caused by outdoor pollutants. In my opinion, the number of cancer cases caused by external pollutants is seriously high. The key here is to minimize exposure and strengthen the body's ability to defend itself against the negative factors in the environment.

Chronic Sunlight Exposure

Our earth's protective barrier from UV rays continues to be compromised. The earth's upper atmosphere has expanded, weakening the earth's natural shield against it. With this weakening comes the increase in the number of skin cancer cases seen each year. There are primarily three forms of skin cancer: melanoma, squamous, and basal cell types. Melanoma is the most lethal type of skin cancer. The number of melanoma cases annually is approximately forty thousand. The other two forms in comparison are approximately seven thousand. Using natural-based protective barrier creams against direct UV rays can minimize the risk of these cancers. Generally speaking, the damaging effects of too much sunlight on fair skin, which can also cause the immune system to be suppressed, can occur years before an actual tumor appears. This cancer risk can be minimized through prevention.

Food Additives

There are many chemicals added to foods to preserve shelf life. These chemicals are also used to enhance palatability of processed foods. There are over three thousand of these chemicals used every year, and many have not been studied for their adverse effects on humans. Some of the most common food additives are:

- saccharin
- cyclamates
- aflatoxins
- aspartame
- hydroxytoluene

These chemicals are known to cause adverse biological activity, which can increase cancer risk significantly. Eating whole foods that are free of preservatives is the key to minimizing this cancer risk and the answer for healthier living.

Free Radicals

Today, we are exposed to all kinds of external and internal factors that can impair our health. Free radicals are among the most potentially harmful agents in existence. A free radical is an unstable molecule with an unpaired electron that steals an electron from another molecule, producing harmful effects. Antioxidants (vitamin A, C, E, selenium, CoQ10, glutathione, and proanthocyanadins) are used to protect against these harmful effects. Free radicals are produced by both external factors (environmental pollution) and internal factors (immune defense and metabolism). Antioxidants can profoundly protect against such negative influences.

Genetic Predisposition

All cancers are genetic in that they are triggered by altered genes. However, just a small portion of cancer is inherited: a mutation carried in reproductive cells, passed on from one generation to the next, and present in cells throughout the body. Most cancers come from random mutations that develop in body cells during one's lifetime—either as a mistake when cells are going through cell division or in response to injuries from environmental agents such as radiation or chemicals. The involvement of genes in cancer is a complex subject. A term that is now used to describe the family tendency for particular cancers is "family cancer syndrome." The term implies that the cancer is likely to show up in succeeding generations of the same family.

Many advances are being made in cancer technology. Many genes are being identified with certain cancer types:

- adenocarcinoma of lung, pancreas, and colon—K-ras

- brain cancer—MSH2, MLH1, PMS1, PMS2

- breast cancer—BRCA1, cyclin D1, erb-B2

- colon and uterine cancer—BRCA2, DCC, K-ras, APC

- endocrine cancer—MEN1, MEN2a

- leukemia—ATM, BLM, FA-A,C

- lung cancer—myc, erb-B2, cyclin D1, abl

- lymphoma—ATM, BLM

- pancreatic cancer—p16, BRCA2, MLH1, MSH2, PMS1, PMS2, K-ras

- skin cancer—p16 (melanoma), BLM

- thyroid cancer—MEN2B

Genetic predisposition doesn't imply that you are going to develop the cancer. It is a term that should inspire you to lead a more health-conscious lifestyle in order to beat the odds of developing cancer.

Heavy Metal Toxicity

Heavy metals, such as mercury, arsenic, nickel, lead, and cadmium are among the most common known to cause dysfunction in the body. These metals accumulate in healthy body tissue, causing toxic symptoms. Some of these symptoms include fatigue, joint aching, difficulty concentrating, headache, impaired bowel function, and cold hands and feet. There are ways to test for concentrations of these heavy metals. Urinary, blood, and hair analysis are available to determine if concentrations of these are increased in the body. In addition, ELISA/ACT testing is available to give a more accurate result on concentration within cells. Consult your physician on your options. Detoxification and chelation therapy may be indicated to help rid your body of these toxic metals, although identifying the source of exposure is essential.

Hormonal Imbalances

Hormonal imbalance can significantly increase cancer risk. There have been studies that have shown the risk of cancer to be higher in women who are using birth control as compared to nonusers.[2] It is essential to determine the underlying cause of hormonal imbalance and to have the appropriate treatment. Hormonal analyses, using blood, urine, and/or saliva are helpful diagnostic tools. There are other treatment options available. Natural hormone therapy and the use of certain herbs and nutrients demonstrate positive benefits. You may want to discuss this with your doctor.

Immune-Suppressing Drugs

There are a great number of conventional drugs, antibiotics, and vaccines that can have suppressive effects on the immune system. Any suppression of the immune system is unfavorable, except in cases of organ transplantation and tissue rejection. In these cases, it is necessary to modulate the immune system to prevent the loss of function. Vaccinations have suppressive effects on the T lymphocytes, which are an integral part of immune defense and regulation. This could set the stage for the onset of chronic disease. Antibiotics hinder immune response and disturb intestinal immune defense by killing off friendly bacteria that protect from potential disease-causing bacteria, viruses, and parasites.

Intestinal Toxicity

Besides the skin, the intestines have the largest surface area contained in the human body. Twenty-five feet of intestine lying out smooth provides approximately two and one-quarter miles of surface area. Many illnesses, including cancer, allergies, and chronic infections can be attributed to toxic bowel function. If the intestines become clogged and diseased, a toxic environment results. Often, an individual with such a toxic bowel is terribly ill. Diet is an essential part of bowel health. Heavy meat eaters and junk-food junkies are ruining their bowels; and over time, they will pay the consequences. Bowel cleansing and detoxification are strongly recommended. Stool digestive analysis is highly advised to determine the health of the bowel. In addition, replenishing healthy bowel bacteria in order to counteract the potentially harmful bacteria is essential. Speak to your doctor about bowel health and how to optimize it.

Oncogenes

In conventional medicine, the emphasis is to find individual genes capable of causing cancerous cells to proliferate and form tumors. Oncogenes were first identified in the 1970s, and currently there are over fifty different oncogenes responsible for specific cancer types. An oncogene is a gene that causes normal cells to behave in a dysfunctional fashion, thus causing the development of cancer. With the new development that comes from the breaking of the genetic code, some new promising cancer therapies can be designed specifically to attack the cancer and spare healthy tissue. Cancer types will be identified genetically, and therapy will be genetically engineered. The positive benefits may include less side reactions to treatment, better quality of life while undergoing treatment, and hope of cure.

Pesticides and Herbicides

The use of pesticides and herbicides is widespread and alarming. Their usage has increased phenomenally since 1945. Over four hundred pesticides are currently licensed for use on our food supply in the US. Approximately 1.5 billion pounds of these thousands of varied chemical compounds and formulations are dumped on crops, forests, lawns, and fields, annually. The Environmental Protection Agency has identified many pesticides and herbicides that could leave carcinogenic residues on foods. These chemicals build up in body tissue and cause toxic accumulation. This process is called "bioaccumulation." Such accumulation in fatty cells (breast, brain, and sexual organs) can initiate cancerous activity. Detoxification and chelation therapy may be necessary to remove these toxic compounds. In addition, careful selection and cleaning of the foods you eat are necessary precautions to assure healthier body function.

Polluted Water

Our water supply in North America is not as pure as it was fifty years ago. There are many organic chemicals and heavy metals found in higher concentrations with each passing decade. It takes greater efforts to purify the water using reverse osmosis and UV filtration. It is important to remember that approximately 75% of the toxins from water that enter the body accumulate in vital tissues. The liver can become overloaded and impaired by these pollutants, which can, in turn, cause cancerous activity to increase. Another problem is the use of chlorine and fluorine, two toxic compounds used to purify water and assure dental hygiene. Both of these elements are known to initiate cancerous activity. It is recommended that purified, filtered water, without the use of chlorine and fluorine, be used. When shopping for pure water, ask for a chemical and biological analysis. In addition, it is important to know where the water source is coming from. This information is available to you without charge. Your water supply should be free of any toxic elements and/or compounds as well as any harmful organisms, such as Giardia and Cryptosporidium, which impair healthy body function.

Tobacco, Smoking, and Alcohol

Tobacco, smoking, and alcohol consumption are among the top cancer causing agents known. It is estimated that 300,000 deaths occur each year in the US as a result of tobacco and alcohol use. There are a variety of cancers that are caused by using tobacco and alcohol:

- pancreatic cancer
- liver cancer
- tongue and lip cancer
- throat cancer
- stomach cancer

- lung cancer

- leukemia

- kidney cancer

- bladder cancer

All cancers caused by cigarette smoking, and heavy use of alcohol could be prevented completely. The American Cancer Society estimates that in the year 2004, 185,000 cancer deaths are expected to be caused by tobacco use, and about twenty-two thousand cancer deaths may be related to excessive alcohol use, frequently in combination with tobacco use. It would be prudent to abstain from the use of tobacco and alcohol in order to promote a healthier lifestyle. The risks far outweigh the benefits and the medical literature proves it.

Viruses

Viruses are non-living particles that look for a living host to replicate. Approximately 15% of the world's cancer cases have been linked to a viral cause. Hepatitis B and C, human papillomavirus (HPV type 16 and 18), Cytomegalovirus (CMV), and Epstein-Barr (EBV), the same virus that causes "mono," are suspect in increasing cancer risk. There are many other viruses that are suspect in causing cancer, including the stealth viruses and the Spuma class of viruses.

CAN CANCER BE PREVENTED OR CURED?

Scientific evidence suggests that about one-third of the 555,500 cancer deaths that occurred in 2002 were related to nutrition and other lifestyle factors. The American Cancer Society estimated in 2002 that 170,000 cancer deaths were caused by tobacco use. Certain cancers are related to viral infections—for example, hepatitis B virus (HBV), human papillomavirus (HPV), human immunodeficiency virus (HIV), human T-cell leukemia/lymphoma virus-I

(HTLV-I), and others—and could be prevented through behavioral and lifestyle changes. In addition, many of the one million skin cancers in the US in 2002 could have been prevented by protection from the sun's rays.

Regular screening examinations by a health care professional can result in the detection of cancers of the breast, colon, rectum, cervix, prostate, testis, oral cavity, and skin at earlier stages, when treatment is more likely to be successful. Self-examinations for cancers of the breast and skin may also result in detection of tumors at earlier stages. The screening-accessible cancers listed above account for about half of all new cancer cases. The five-year relative survival rate for these cancers is about 80%. If all Americans participated in regular cancer screenings, this rate could increase to 95%.

WHO IS AT RISK OF DEVELOPING CANCER?

Anyone. Aging is considered a risk factor; most cases affect adults middle-aged or older. Nearly 80% of all cancers are diagnosed at ages fifty-five and older. Cancer researchers use the word *risk* in different ways. *Lifetime risk* refers to the probability that an individual, over the course of a lifetime, will develop cancer or die from it. In the US, men have a one in two lifetime risk of developing cancer; for women, the risk is one in three.

Relative risk is a measure of the strength of the relationship between risk factors and the particular cancer. It compares the risk of developing cancer in persons with a certain exposure or trait to the risk in persons who do not have this exposure or trait. For example, smokers have a ten-fold relative risk of developing lung cancer compared with nonsmokers. This means that smokers are about ten times more likely to develop lung cancer (or have a 900% increased risk) than nonsmokers. Most relative risks are not this large. For example, women who have a first-degree (mother, sister, or daughter) family history of breast cancer have about a two-fold increased risk of developing breast cancer compared with women who do not have a family history. This means that women with a first-degree family history are about two times or 100% more likely to develop breast cancer than women who do not have a family history of the disease.

All cancers involve the malfunction of genes that control cell growth and division. About 5 to 10% of cancers are clearly hereditary, in that an inherited faulty gene predisposes the person to a very high risk of particular cancers. The remainder of cancers is not hereditary but results from damage to genes (mutations) that occurs throughout our lifetime, either due to internal factors, such as hormones or the digestion of nutrients within cells, or to external factors, such as chemicals and sunlight.

How Many People Alive Today Have Had Cancer?

The National Cancer Institute estimates that approximately 8.9 million Americans alive today have a history of cancer. Some of these individuals can be considered cured, while others still have evidence of cancer and may be undergoing treatment. The ability to determine the number of active cases of cancer raises global awareness of the disease. The occurrence of cancer continues to rise because of environmental, genetics, and lifestyle factors.

How Many New Cases Are Expected to Occur This Year?

About 1.3 million new cancer cases are forecasted in 2004. Since 1990, according to the American Cancer Society, approximately 16 million new cancer cases have been diagnosed. These estimates do not include carcinoma in situ (noninvasive cancer) of any site, except urinary bladder, and do not include basal and squamous cell skin cancers. In 2004 a forecast of approximately 1.4 million cases of basal and squamous cell skin cancers are expected to occur.

How Many People Are Expected to Die of Cancer This Year?

In 2002 the American Cancer Society estimated 555,500 American deaths related to cancer—more than 1,500 people a day. Cancer is the second leading cause of death in the US, exceeded only by heart disease. In the US, one of every four deaths is from cancer.

What Percentage of People Survive Cancer?

Five-year relative survival rates are commonly used to monitor progress in the early detection and treatment of cancer. The *relative survival rate* is the survival rate observed for a group of cancer patients compared to the survival rate for persons in the general population who are similar to the patient group with respect to age, gender, race, and calendar year of observation. Relative survival adjusts for normal life expectancy (factors such as dying of heart disease, accidents, and diseases of old age).

Five-year relative survival rates include persons who are living five years after diagnosis, whether in remission, disease-free, or under treatment. While these rates provide some indication about the average survival experience of cancer patients in a given population, they are less informative when used to predict individual prognosis and should be interpreted with caution. First, five-year relative survival rates are based on patients who were diagnosed and treated at least eight years ago and do not reflect recent advances in treatment. Second, information about detection methods, treatment protocols, additional illnesses, and behaviors that influence survival are not taken into account in the estimation of survival rates. The five-year relative survival rate for all cancers combined is 59%.

Sometimes, patients use statistics to try to figure out their chance of being cured. It is important to remember, however, that statistics are averages based on large numbers of patients.

They cannot be used to predict what will happen to a particular patient because no two patients are alike. The doctor who takes care of the patient is in the best position to discuss the chance of recovery (prognosis). Patients should feel free to ask the doctor about their prognosis, but they should keep in mind that not even the doctor knows exactly what will happen. Doctors often talk about surviving cancer, or they may use the term "remission," rather than "cure." Even though many cancer patients are cured, doctors use "remission," because the disease may recur.

I believe it crucial to mention that an individual's focus should be on healing and not the negative aspects of the prognosis. I encourage my patients to focus on their healing and not their disease process. Focusing upon healing heightens the body's chance of recovery and also energizes the fight for the precious gift of life. This is not denial that the disease exists; it is simply refocusing and transforming the disease process into wellness.

STAGING OF CANCER?

The staging of cancer is specific for the cancer types. In this paragraph the staging of cancer is described in general terms. In the next chapter, discussion of staging to the particular type of cancer is given. According to the American Cancer Society, staging is the process of describing the extent of the disease or the spread of cancer from the site of origin. Staging is essential in determining the choice of therapy and assessing prognosis. A cancer's stage is based on information about the primary tumor's size and location in the body and whether or not it has spread to other areas of the body.

A number of different staging systems are currently being used to classify tumors. The TNM staging system assesses tumors in three ways: extent of the primary tumor (T), absence or presence of regional lymph node involvement (N), and absence or presence of distant metastases (M). Once the T, N, and M are determined, a "stage" of I, II, III, or IV is assigned, with stage I being early stage and IV being advanced stage. Summary staging (in situ, local, regional, and distant) has been useful for descriptive and statistical analysis of tumor registry data. If cancer cells are present only in the layer of cells they developed in, and they have not spread to other parts of that organ or elsewhere in the body, then the stage is in situ. If cancer cells have spread beyond the original layer of tissue, then the cancer is considered invasive. In the next chapter on common cancers, discussion of staging is more specific to the type of cancer.

WHAT ARE THE COSTS OF CANCER?

The National Institutes of Health estimates overall annual costs for cancer at $115 billion: $45 billion for direct medical costs (total of all health expenditures), $11 billion for indirect morbidity costs (cost of lost productivity due to illness), and $59 billion for indirect mortality costs (cost of lost productivity due to premature death). Treatment of breast, lung, and prostate cancers account for over half of the direct medical costs and are among the most common cancers in the US. Insurance status and barriers to health care may affect the cost of treating cancer in this country. According to 1996 data, about 19% of Americans under age sixty-five have no health insurance, and about 26% of older persons have only Medicare coverage. During 1996, almost 18% of Americans reported not having a usual source of health care. Also, 12% of American families had members who experienced difficulty or delay in obtaining care or did not receive needed health care services.

Chapter 5

Commonly Treated Cancers

Cancer has been present throughout human history. Egyptian and Incan mummies show evidence of the disorder. Greek physicians described it, and Hippocrates provided its name. However, accurate information regarding the occurrence of cancer has been captured only within the last century.

—American Cancer Society

I n this chapter there will be definitions and information on the most common cancers. With all the current information on cancer, it would take several volumes to adequately cover every type of cancer in existence today. For the sake of space, discussion on the most prevalent cancers, with information that is pertinent to understanding the diagnosis, treatment, and outcome, is covered in this chapter. Any further inquiries should be directed to the American Cancer Society, National Institute of Health, or other reputable sources. The following is a list of what will be discussed:

- bladder cancer
- breast cancer

- gynecological cancers (uterine and ovarian)
- leukemia
- lung cancer
- lymphoma
- melanoma
- pancreatic cancer
- prostate cancer
- rectal and colon (bowel) cancer

BLADDER CANCER

An estimated 270,000 new cases of bladder cancer occur annually, with fifty-three thousand of them occurring in the United States. Bladder cancer is considered the fourth most prevalent malignancy in the United States. Bladder cancer is divided into superficial and invasive disease. Improvements in current treatment regimens have improved quality of life in individuals with invasive disease.

Some of the potential risk factors include:

- continuous exposure to organic chemicals of petroleum origin
- cigarette smoke and chewing tobacco
- decreased water intake
- pesticides
- chronic bladder infections
- heavy metal exposure

Current Staging of Bladder Cancer

"Transitional cell carcinoma" is the term used in cancer medicine to describe the progression of the disease. The following staging classification is used to assist you in understanding the areas effected by the cancer:

- Tis—carcinoma in situ

- Ta—tumors not invading the lamina propria

- T1—tumors invading the lamina propria

- T2a—tumors that invade the detrusor muscle

- T2b—tumors that invade the deeper layers of the detrusor muscle

- T3—tumors that extend into the perivesical fat

- T3a micro—tumors are visualized microscopically

- T3b macro—tumors are visualized without the use of microscope

- T4—tumors invade adjacent structures (prostate, uterus or vagina, pelvic, or abdominal side wall)

The most common sign of bladder cancer is blood in the urine. Usually, passing of blood in the urine is painless and intermittent. This can be accompanied by urinary frequency, urgency, or inability to urinate. If any of these symptoms appear, it is necessary to have them checked by your physician.

There are laboratory markers found in the urine that can be used to screen those who are in high-risk categories. The most valuable diagnostic tool is cystoscopic examination, intravenous urography, and urinary cytology. In some cases an MRI is useful in identifying the extent of tumor growth.

In summary, bladder cancer is a common malignancy, and its incidence continues to increase due to exposure to environmental carcinogens and tobacco. Prompt and appropriate diagnosis of the source of blood in the urine can reduce the stage of the disease significantly and improve survival rates. Options in treatment are BCG immunotherapy (depends upon staging), chemotherapy (usually Taxol® or gemcitabine), combined radiation and chemotherapy, resection of bladder, and/or removal of bladder. Removal of the bladder is not the first course of action and should not be considered as a first treatment option. See the bladder cancer case discussed in chapter fifteen for a sample plan of integrative treatment that demonstrated a great outcome. In appendix six, a general, oral, natural medicine regimen is listed. In appendices one and two, there is a sample list of chemo agents and regimens used in bladder cancer.

BREAST CANCER

Breast cancer is the most common type of malignant tumor among women of the Western world. Approximately 182,800 new cases will be diagnosed in American women in 2003. The incidence of the disease increased between 1940 and 1987. Between 1982 and 1986, the rate increased by 4% per year, but since 1987, the incidence rate has been relatively stable. Breast cancer mortality has been stable since 1950, although mortality has increased among women older than fifty-five years and has decreased among women younger than fifty-five. To a certain extent, the stable mortality and increasing incidence may reflect an increase in the rate at which carcinoma in situ and small, occult, invasive cancers are being discovered as a result of more widespread use of mammography, or it may indicate a more fundamental change in incidence. Finally, improvements in treatment may have contributed to an increase in the percentage of breast cancers that have been cured over the last thirty years.

These raw statistics mask the broader emotional and financial impact of the disease. For every woman with a diagnosis of breast cancer, another five or ten will have a biopsy that shows benign disease. For every woman who undergoes biopsy, perhaps ten or more see their physician because of a breast symptom and concern about cancer or have a cancer question raised by an abnormal mammogram.

Risk Factors for Developing Breast Cancer

Lifetime risk for American women for breast cancer is measured on a scale from birth-110 years and demonstrates about 13%, but the risk from dying from the cancer is 3.3%.

Hereditary factors:

- familial

- genetic

Prior history of breast cancer:

- benign breast disease (atypical hyperplasia)

- in situ

- invasive

Endogenous endocrine factors:

- age at menarche

- age at menopause

- age at first pregnancy

Exogenous endocrine factors:

- postmenopausal estrogen replacement

- oral contraceptives

Environmental factors:

- region of birth

- diet

- alcohol

Staging

Staging of breast cancer is necessary in determining prognosis and the form of treatment that is most effective. The staging system that is used currently is the TNM system (T=tumor, N=node, and M=metastasis). Physical examination and mammography are used to determine staging. In addition, lymph nodes may need a biopsy to determine the spread of the disease. This lymph node sampling may be necessary to determine the specific therapy with the most effective outcome.

In patients who have positive nodes, one large study has concluded that at least ten axillary lymph nodes should be evaluated to separate those in a low-risk group (i.e., fewer than four positive nodes) from those in a high-risk group (i.e., four or more positive nodes). The incidence of arm edema or other complications is related to the extent of the axillary surgery. When the dissection is limited to nodal tissue lateral to the pectoralis minor muscle, the risk of such complications is low. Sentinel node biopsy is an attempt to establish the status of the axillary lymph nodes while limiting the risk of arm edema.

Note: In many patients with breast cancer I have treated, I have observed edema, even with sentinel node dissection. My patients have received lymphatic drainage massage and intravenous nutritional support as well as homeopathic drainage support.

Prognosis

In prognosis, tumor size and lymph node involvement are at this time the best predictive factors. The ten-year survival rate in patients without nodal involvement is about 65–70%. Nodal spread decreases the survival rate. However, focusing on prognosis alone can lead to poor outcomes because the emphasis is on the disease process rather than the healing power of the body. Empowerment alone can be the strongest healing element, and I believe that sharing this with my patients fighting the battle against cancer is crucial. In cases of noninvasive carcinoma of the breast, the ten-year survival rate is higher and prognosis is excellent.

See the breast cancer case discussed in chapter fifteen for a sample plan of integrative treatment that demonstrated a great outcome. In appendix six, a general, oral, natural medicine regimen is listed. In appendices one and two, there is a sample list of chemo agents and regimens used in breast cancer.

GYNECOLOGICAL CANCERS (CERVICAL, VAGINAL, VULVAR, UTERINE, AND OVARIAN)

Tumors of the female reproductive tract include cancers of the vulva, vagina, cervix, uterus, fallopian tubes, and ovaries. These tumors represent approximately 13.4% of all cancers affecting women and account for 10% of their cancer deaths. It is essential for doctors to adequately screen for these cancers because early detection improves the outcomes. There are many risk factors associated with these cancer types, which include sexually transmitted agents, viral (HSV and HPV), genetic influences, lifestyle influences, hormonal factors, etc. Early detection through the use of Pap smear, utilizing Papnet, Accupap, or Autopap technology, can significantly reduce false negatives and improve overall detection statistics.

It is very important to have annual exams for early detection of disease for all of these gynecological cancers.

Diagnosis

In cases of cervical, vulva, and vaginal cancer, the starting place is the use of Pap-enhanced, cell-reading technology. In cancer of the uterus, Pap and pelvic exam, imaging, and biopsy may be used. In ovarian tumors, the screening cancer marker CA125 should be part of the diagnostic work-up, along with diagnostic imaging (ultrasound, MRI, and/or CT scan. Other diagnostic tests, procedures, and biopsy may be indicated to establish a diagnosis. It is essential to stay informed throughout the process and consult either the Internet resources like the American Cancer Society and/or National Institute of Health (NIH) Cancer Library.

Staging

In screening cervical cancer, the CIN, Pap classification, and Bethesda system are all staging systems in use, currently. In addition, if a lesion is detected, the TNM system is used. The TNM system is also used in vulvar and vaginal cancer. For a description of TNM for each of the above gynecological cancers, consult the American Cancer Society and/or NIH information, either on the Internet or in their publications.

Treatment

Conventional treatment includes chemotherapy, radiation therapy, cryosurgery, geneal surgery, immunotherapy, and hormonal and anti-hormonal therapy. Each of these forms of treatment, depending on the type of cancer, can be used. Integrative treatment is highly recommended for better outcomes. See appendix for more information.

LEUKEMIA

In the United States, leukemias account for approximately 3% of all cancers and 4% of all cancer deaths. The leukemias are divided into two categories: acute and chronic. In acute leukemia, there is increased proliferation of immature cells and impaired differentiation. If untreated, this form can be fatal in weeks to months. In chronic leukemia, there is increased proliferation, but cells are able to mature and differentiate. Generally, chronic leukemias have an indolent course.

The leukemias are divided further into subtypes including lymphoid, myeloid, and bisphenotypic, which are defined by the predominant leukemic cell population. Advances in both the treatment and supportive therapies have led to an improvement in the outcomes for both acute and chronic leukemias.

Diagnosis

Blood testing, bone marrow testing, and cytogenetic evaluation are essential in determining the diagnosis. Immunophenotyping may also be used to distinguish between different subtypes.

Staging

Staging is based on physical findings and laboratory evaluation, which may include cytogenic and immunogenic evaluation.

Treatment

Treatment varies with the subtype of leukemia. Treatments can include conventional chemotherapy, radiation therapy, bone marrow transplantation, immunothrapy, and possible genetic therapy.

Summary

The leukemias can effect all ages. The application in the latest technological advances allows for better detection and classification. The application of new molecular and genetic advances has aided in better classification and treatment of both acute and chronic leukemias. New therapies have changed the prognosis and outcomes. Over the last ten years, the outcomes of patients diagnosed with leukemia have changed from uniformly fatal to potentially curable. Again, it is important to consider integrative therapy in combination with traditional therapies to facilitate a curative outcome. See the appendix in the back of the book for integrative treatments, and consult your physician specialist of integrative medicine.

LUNG CANCER

Lung cancer is of major concern for the Public Health Department. According to the latest figures, more than 150,000 deaths occur annually in the United States. The major contributor to lung cancer is the use of tobacco. This cancer can significantly reduce in numbers by simply eliminating the usage of tobacco. Cigarette smoking constitutes the greatest risk factor in the development of lung cancer. Other less common risk factors include exposures to heavy metals, including arsenic, chromium, and nickel. In addition, ionizing radiation, vinyl chloride, chlormethyl ether, and polycyclic aromatic hydrocarbons are included as less common causes of lung cancer. Preexisting lung diseases such as pulmonary fibrosis and chronic obstructive lung diseases are also considered risk factors in developing lung cancer.

Epidemiological studies demonstrate a reduction in lung cancer risk in individuals who consume large amounts of fruits and vegetables. This is due to the increased levels of antioxidants, including beta-carotene, vitamin A, and other antioxidants. It is essential to consider diet and other important nutrients that demonstrate protection against cancer.

A common genetic abnormality in lung cancer is the loss of 3p. This abnormality is demonstrated in small-cell lung carcinoma (SCLC) and non-small-cell carcinoma (NSCLC). Several regions of this chromosome are altered. In addition to the loss of chromosome 3p, there seems to be a similar pattern of loss on chromosomes 5, 9, 13, and 17, as well as other sites. This all points to strong evidence of hereditary and environmental influences, causing mutations to occur from generation to generation.

There is also known *p53* mutations that occur in lung cancer. Other expressions include HER-2/*neu* and *ras* gene. These markers usually indicate poor outcomes, particularly with regards to adenocarcinoma.

Different Classifications of Lung Cancer

1. Small-Cell Lung Cancer (SCLC)—SCLC represents approximately 20–30% of all cases of lung cancer. Current classification by WHO designates three subtypes, which include Oat-cell carcinoma, small-cell carcinoma, and combined oat-cell carcinoma. Little evidence suggests that these subtypes have prognostic value.

2. Non-Small-Cell Lung Cancer (NSCLC)—NSCLC represent approximately 10-15% of all lung cancers. They tend to occur on the periphery of the lung, invading bronchi and larger airways.

3. Squamous Cell Carcinoma—There is a steady decline in the prevalence of this type of lung cancer. There is no clear determination as to why this cancer is on the decline. Maybe greater awareness to healthier living is contributing to the decline.

4. Adenocarcinoma—Adenocarcinoma is the most common subtype of lung cancer in the United States, representing 40-50% of all lung cancers. In general, adenocarcinoma has the worst prognosis of all the subtypes.

5. Carcinoid Tumor of the Lung—These tumors are uncommon. They have their origin in the neuroendocrine system responsible for hormonal signaling, which may account for the carcinoid tumor to develop.

Diagnosis

Various forms of imaging that may include CT scanning, PET scanning, MRI and diagnostic procedures that include bronchoscopy may be necessary. Biopsy is taken and analyzed to determine subtype.

Staging

The TNM classification of staging is used with some variation. The staging in lung subtypes varies and can be quite difficult to understand. Detailed discussion with your oncologist is recommended to gain a better understanding of staging.

Treatment

Treatment can include traditional chemotherapy and radiation therapy. Sometimes surgical excision of the tumor can be performed, if the tumor is operable. For advanced stage IV with brain metastasis, the outcomes are not medically favorable. Gamma knife radiosurgery may be a viable option. It is so important to consider integrative treatment options available. Intravenous nutrient therapy with trace mineral and antioxidant support can be highly beneficial. Considering autologous vaccine with immune modulating properties is also recommended. Dietary and lifestyle goals are very important. Spirit and soul healing is essential for better outcomes. See appendix for sample treatments and sample prayer in the section the journey toward healing.

LYMPHOMA (HODGKIN'S DISEASE OR NON-HODGKIN'S LYMPHOMA [NHL])

One of the key signs of development of a lymphoma is persistent, unexplained, swollen lymph glands. Additional symptoms that might accompany this: fever, chills, night sweats, unexplained weight loss, and general unexplained itching. Hodgkin's disease is different from non-Hodgkin's lymphoma on the basis of cause, disease process, progression of disease in the body in the lymph nodes, and particularly, response to treatment and overall outcome.

Hodgkin's Disease (HD)

Hodgkin's presents itself generally in painless, swollen lymph nodes accompanied by fever, chills, night sweats, itching, and weight loss. In addition, there may be pain in a lymph node-bearing area, associated with the consumption of alcohol. HD accounts for 14% of lymphomas. The cause of HD is unknown, and there is increased suspicion that toxic environmental exposures cause the disease. Agricultural workers, farmers, meat workers, and woodworkers have had an increase of HD. Individuals with a history of infectious mononucleosis (mono caused by EBV) have a threefold chance in developing the disease. Viruses, including Epstein Barr Virus (EBV), HIV, and others that may include cytomegalovirus (CMV), and SPUMA class viruses are also suspect in causing the disease. Further research is being conducted to establish viral causes.

> **Diagnosis:** Diagnosis of HD is achieved by a needle aspiration or a lymph node biopsy. The distinctive cell type in HD is the Reed-Sternberg cell, which contains EBV DNA, which is why EBV is strongly suspected as a cause of the disease. Cytogenetic and molecular genetic studies may also be part of the diagnostic work-up. There are different classifications of the disease proposed by WHO, and, for further information regarding classification, consult either the American Cancer Society (ACS) or NIH sources.

> **Staging:** The four-stage clinical and pathologic Ann Arbor system has been widely used for the last twenty-five years. For a description of this, consult ACS and/or NIH information. To determine extent of involvement of the disease, various forms of imaging are done, including chest X-ray, SPECT scans, CT of abdomen and pelvic region, PET scan, and MRI. In some cases, bone marrow biopsy may be also used.

Treatment: Conventional treatments include chemotherapy (ABVD, Stanford V, BEACOPP) and radiation therapy. Bone marrow transplantation has not
demonstrated favorable outcomes at this time and
is still being evaluated. Other treatment options are
being explored. Integrative therapies are definitely
helpful in increasing the remission rate. HD is considered either completely or partially remitted with
conventional treatment. With radiation therapy in
early stage disease, complete remission is achieved.
Failure free survival rate for a twenty-year period
and beyond is 75–90%. Relapses of the disease do
occur in 20–30% of patients previously treated with
conventional treatment and 20–30% never achieve
complete or partial remission.

Non-Hodgkin's Lymphoma (NHL)

NHL is the fifth most common tumor type diagnosed in men
in the United States each year and the sixth in women. The age
range in which this cancer occurs can be from twenty-eight to
sixty-five years of age, depending upon the subtype. The cause
of NHL is unknown presently. However, as is the case for HD
with NHL, there is increased suspicion that environmental exposure and virus exposure is the cause. The HIV, HTLV-1, and
HHV-8 are suspected viruses, and further research is being conducted on other viruses that may cause the disease. There are
genetic changes that occur in NHL and continued research re-
veals definite genetic influences in disease process.

Diagnosis: A biopsy or needle aspiration of the involved
lymph node. Cytogenetic and molecular genetic
studies may also be part of the diagnostic work-up.
WHO has classification standards for NHL, and either ACS or NIH information sources should be con-
sulted for specific information.

Staging: The Ann Arbor is also used in NHL but is less relevant than in HD, because NHL exhibits more advanced spread of the disease at presentation of the disease process. Special imaging procedures may be required to determine staging of the disease. The imaging methods used are similar to HD.

Treatment: The current approach to treatment of NHL varies with the stage and subtype. Radiation therapy is the treatment of choice with an overall ten-year survival rate of approximately 50–80%. However, this all depends on accurate staging of the disease. Chemotherapy and radiation therapy have been used in combination. New immunotherapeutic and biological class agents are demonstrating promising results. Stem cell transplantation continues to be under investigation. Currently, Bone Marrow Transplantation (BMT), as reported by the BMT Registry, shows that, of eighty-one patients transplanted at an age of forty years of age, 56% never achieved a complete remission. The death rate from BMT is an overall 44%, and it was usually the chemotherapy sensitivity that caused the deaths to occur. It is vital that treatment options be explored carefully. Always remember that empowerment is the key. If you feel forced by medical professionals, friends, or family members into making a decision regarding treatment, that is the first mistake!

Integrative medicine in combination with conventional treatment increases health and vitality during treatment while enhancing the body's ability to heal. Autologous vaccine should be considered in NHL. For an outline of recommended integrative treatment options, consult the appendix.

Melanoma

Melanomas develop by a malignant transformation of the melanocyte. This is a skin cell that is responsible for the healthy protection of the skin to harmful influences like UV radiation. Melanoma is often caused by overexposure to the sun. However, there are genetic and familial patterns in the disease process. The current five-year survival rate is approximately 88%, which is a marked improvement over the last thirty years. Melanoma accounts for 4% of all cancers in the United States. The incidence of this cancer continues to increase. It is important to watch certain types of skin moles for change in appearance and/or color, because these may be suspicious for melanoma. Prevention is to limit sun exposure and to use protective sunscreens. However, there have been reports of sunscreens actually increasing the risk by allowing susceptible individuals to remain out in the direct sun for longer periods of time without developing a burn. Tanning beds can contribute to increase risk, but an exact account is not determined at this time. It is essential that you use common sense with regard to sun exposure. Protect your skin and you will reduce the risk!

Diagnosis

Diagnosis is made by biopsy of the suspicious lesion. If there are changes in a mole that include color, growth, borders, itching, and/or bleeding, then these need to biopsied. There are four common growth patterns in melanoma, and this is distinguished by studying the cell growth patterns.

Staging

Clinical staging of primary tumors is extremely inaccurate, both in terms of estimating the thickness of the primary tumor and of judging the spread of the disease. Biopsy and pathological interpretation are the crucial elements in establishing a diagnosis and staging of the disease. Currently, the TNM system is used in staging the disease process. Special imaging procedures may be done to determine the spread of the disease and this is case-determined.

Treatment

Treatment depends upon the staging of the disease. Removal of the lesions is usually the treatment of choice. If spread of the disease is suspected, then a sentinel node biopsy may be the next step to identify if the disease spread to the nearby lymph nodes. Chemotherapy, biological therapy, and immunotherapy are considerations for treatment of the disease. Vaccines with the use of IL-2 and IL-12 have been used with response rates of up to 40% in metastatic disease. Gene therapy is being evaluated. Brain metastases have been treated with gamma-knife therapy more successfully as compared to traditional radiotherapy. In comparison, gamma-knife recipients had median survival rates up to thirty-five weeks, as compared to four to six weeks with conventional radiation. Integrative treatment, including autologous vaccine with IL-12, is recommended as an adjuvant treatment regimen.

PANCREATIC CANCER

Higher incidences of pancreatic cancer have been seen within the last ten years. A resulting 22% of all cancer-related deaths is caused by pancreatic cancer. Overall, pancreatic cancer is the fourth leading cause of cancer in both men and women. The ability to diagnose and improve the cure rates is difficult because of the position of the pancreas in the body and the usual late presentation of the disease. More particulars about guidelines on diagnosing and managing this disease can be found on the web site *www.nccn.org*.

The majority of the cases of pancreatic cancer occur in individuals between the ages of sixty and eighty years old. Pancreatic cancer occurs more frequently in men than in women, but the incidence and death rates have decreased in men while increasing

in women over the last twenty years. Risk factors include hereditary factors, socioeconomic status, habitation of industrialized so-
cieties, environmental and dietary factors, excessive alcohol use,
and cigarette smoking.

Genetically, there are several genetic alterations, including *K-ras, p53, p16, DPC4,* and *BRCA2.* Genetic testing is becoming readily
accepted and will be a valuable part of screening and diagnosis.

Diagnosis

Special imaging that may include CT of the pancreas specifically, MRI, and MRI cholangiopancreatography, ERCP (endoscopic retrograde cholangiopancreatography), and Endoscopic
ultrasound. These forms of imaging may be used in combination to locate masses within the pancreas. Another valuable
tool is the use of the cancer marker CA 19-9, which is superior
to other markers because it is more specific to the pancreas.
Elevation of Ca 19-9 yields a positive predictive value of > 99%
when combined with CT imaging of the pancreas. This marker
should be used in combination with imaging. Ca 19-9 can also
be used to monitor response to treatment.

Staging

The TNM staging system is used in pancreatic cancer.

Treatment

Surgical removal of lesion, if operable, with stent placement to
keep the bile channels open is a standard recommendation.
Conventional chemotherapy and radiotherapy may also be recommended. A promising treatment of combined an artemesia
and autologous vaccine has demonstrated favorable results in
decreasing pain, reducing tumor size, and increasing quality of
life in the individual. Integrative therapy is strongly recommended.

Prostate Cancer

Prostate cancer is considered the second leading cause of cancer-related deaths in men. The use of screening blood testing in the form of PSA (prostate specific antigen), physical exam, and ultrasound with biopsy has significantly improved the outcome of prostate cancer in most recent years. Prostate cancer, generally speaking, is slow growing and rarely manifests as an aggressive disease. However, in some cases there can be aggressive disease. Most commonly, men over the age of forty-five should be screened for prostate cancer using PSA and physical exam. I have seen cases of prostate cancer in men who were slightly over fifty years of age. In these cases, catching them early and administering appropriate treatment is essential in decreasing mortality.

Genetically, prostate cancer is complex and involves the androgen receptor gene and p53. Continued research is needed to gain a clearer picture of what is specifically involved. There aren't any specific genetic tests at this time that will give a reliable detection of prostate cancer. Most often time prostate cancer is diagnosed by an onset of symptoms that include urinary difficulties (hesitation, urgency, decreased force, and increased frequency).

Diagnosis

The first important step in detection and diagnosis is digital rectal exam of the prostate gland in combination with a PSA blood test. If PSA is elevated and troublesome findings on digital exam are found, then the next step is transrectal ultrasonography (TRUS). TRUS is accompanied by a six-core biopsy of the prostate gland at the left and right base, midportion, and apex. It is important that all of these areas be studied if suspicion of cancer is high. In some cases, PSA may not be elevated, but trouble symptoms and a positive nodule digital exam will require TRUS and a biopsy to be sure that the prostate is clear. Recently, I have had two cases where PSA values were normal but symptoms and digital exam demonstrated worrisome findings. I sent both patients for TRUS and biopsy and both of them came back with positive cancer in three locations in the prostate with a significant Gleason score.

MRI and bone scanning may be other forms of imaging to determine the extent of the spread of the cancer.

Staging

The American Joint Committee on Cancer TNM (tumor, node, metastasis) staging system is used. In addition, a Gleason grading of the tumor is used to determine the type of growth pattern, which is on a scale of 1–3. PSA, clinical staging, and Gleason score are all required to give a total points axis to determine the prediction of remaining recurrence-free for sixty months.

Treatment

There are a variety of treatments for prostate cancer, including conventional chemotherapy and radiation therapy. In addition, other forms of therapy in certain staging, which include proton therapy and brachytherapy (seed implantation), may be treatments of choice. In some cases, a combination of low-dose chemotherapy used for sensitization with high-energy radiotherapy may be employed. There are cases that require surgical removal, but this should never be the first course.

There are a variety of herbal therapies that include the use of Artemesia, high dose saw palmetto extract, and PC-SPES formulation to inhibit the neoplastic growth. There are also some anti-hormone and immune therapies that may be viable options. Several potential curative options are available and the most invasive forms of intervention should always be the last course. Both patients I mentioned earlier are doing well. Combined integrative therapy was the treatment of choice, and the results were favorable.

Summary

Prostate cancer can be treated successfully. Early detection and treatment utilizing a combined approach is recommended. It is essential that all of your treatment options are explored and that you consider consulting with an integrative medical specialist before making any definite treatment choices. Knowledge, and the correct use of it, dispels confusion and reduces the risk of harm. See appendix for integrative treatment recommendations.

RECTAL AND COLON (BOWEL) CANCER

Colorectal cancer in the United States accounts for 14% of total cancer deaths. It is a disease that effects people fifty years of age and older. The overall five-year cancer survival rate is 62%, with the incidence of death decreasing over the last fifty years. This is due to more accurate screening, diagnosis, and treatment of the disease. Risk factors of the disease include genetic factors, hereditary factors, chronic inflammatory disease, environmental and dietary factors, and psychoemotional factors. There are preventive nutrients that have demonstrated some significant reduction of colorectal cancer incidence, including micronutrients, calcium, and the vitamin folic acid. For example, in one study, folic acid supplements were given at 400 mg/day and ingested over a period of ten to fifteen years, reducing the cancer risk by 50%. Wholesome dietary practices are also important in reducing this risk.

Genetically, MSH2 and MLH1 are involved as well as tumor necrosis factor. K-ras mutation is observed along with DCC loss on chromosome 18q and p53 loss on chromosome 17p. In addition, mutation in the APC gene on chromosome 5 is commonly seen in familial adenomatous polyps, which can predispose to cancer. This new understanding of genetic influences for colon rectal cancer will allow for early diagnosis and improved treatment.

Diagnosis

Routine stool tests for blood in combination with a rectal exam are the starting place for screening. A colonoscopy should be performed at fifty years of age. If there are troublesome symptoms and signs of disease, a colonoscopy should be performed sooner. If there is a family history of colorectal cancer, then screening should begin at age forty.

Staging

The staging criteria for bowel cancer depends upon the examination of the removed diseased tissue from the colon or rectum. The TNM (tumor, node, metastasis) system is the current criteria used in staging colorectal cancer.

Treatment

A variety of treatment options are implemented, including surgery, radiotherapy, chemotherapy, biological therapy, and immune therapy. Autologous vaccine therapy, combined with other integrative treatment, has demonstrated excellent outcomes. Be sure to consult with your integrative medical specialist in order to discover what is available.

KEEP A HOPEFUL OUTLOOK!

The most important message that one can get with regards to cancer diagnosis is to never lose hope and always remember that healing occurs on many levels. Searching out your treatment is vital. Allowing for spiritual and soul healing is vital to the healing process overall. Diagnosis should never mean defeat. People beat the odds all of the time. Miracles happen everyday.

Don't feel pressured into just any form of treatment. Do some homework first and have other trusted individuals help you with this. Establish a family altar of prayer and devotion to God and ask for guidance. Do not discount the possibility of combining integrative therapy, for the benefits are tremendous. Most of all, life is a gift given to you by God, and it deserves every bit of fight you've got! There is no room for lost hope! A good promise to take hold of is found in the biblical Psalm of David: "Why art thou cast down, O my soul? And why art thou disquieted within me? hope in God: for I shall yet praise him, who is the health of my countenance, and my God" (Psalm 43:5). What a great promise coming from a devoted follower of God who realized that every good and perfect gift comes from Him.

● ●

Chapter 6

Cancer Detection and Prevention

Prevention is the most important cancer-fighting tool in existence today.

Prevention requires preparedness—The only king to insure himself against the loss of his throne was Prajadhipok, King of Siam from 1925 until he was forced to abdicate in 1935. Having taken out unemployment insurance policies with French and British underwriters early in his reign, Prajadhipok was able to live comfortably on the income from them until his death in 1941.

—Selected

Cancer prevention should become a way of life, though there are some cancer risks we cannot avoid. The most essential part of prevention is preparedness. Preparedness is actively gathering knowledge and carefully working through the decision-making process in order to avoid potential dangers. In other words, you are not going to just take an expert opinion or recommendation at face value. Early detection of cancer should be part of overall prevention. There are many cancer detection and prevention tests available. Some of these tests are discussed below.

CANCER DETECTION TESTS

AMAS (Anti-Malignant Antibody in Serum)

AMAS is used for the early detection of breast and prostate cancer. A positive AMAS test indicates that cancer tissue is present in the tissue tested. AMAS is an excellent adjunct to other routine detection testing. AMAS is considered ninety-five percent reliable, except in advanced cases of cancer. It is important to remember that testing is always variable, and the more accurate it is, the more likely it will detect more precisely. For more information about AMAS testing contact: *ONCOLAB at 1.800.922.8378.* Licensed physicians can order this test. There are limitations of this test because it may be too sensitive and pick up activity that is not considered cancerous.

Bone Marrow Aspiration

Bone marrow aspiration, or BMA, is a diagnostic test that analyzes the bone marrow. This test is done when cancer of the bone marrow and blood is suspected. It is also used to monitor response to Bone Marrow Transplantation. The procedure is invasive and often painful. It can be done under a general anesthetic, which cuts down on the pain of the procedure. In fact, I recommend my cancer patients have it done under general anesthetic. The marrow is extracted from the hip and the procedure generally takes about ten to thirty minutes. Cytogenetic studies can be performed on the marrow sample if requested by the oncologist or hematologist. I recommend that this be done in order to demonstrate the genetic activity of the cancer. However, in some cases, cytogenetic evaluation is not necessary.

Bone Scan

This is specialized imaging for determining cancerous activity in the bone. A bone scan is usually performed using radionuclide techniques. Technetium 99m-labled phosphonates are used to determine abnormalities in bone and joints. The radio-nuclides are used to minimize the radiation exposure to the patient and are much more specific than X-rays. A bone scan continues to be the preferred diagnostic imaging to determine if a cancer is active in bone.

BTA (Biological Terrain Assessment)

BTA analyzes an individual's internal environment. This test examines blood, urine, and saliva, and evaluates three criteria: pH (acid-base balance), oxidation/reduction potential, and re-sistance. For cancer patients, the test provides more detailed insight into the biochemistry and a more specific treatment plan can be initiated. BTA is by no means diagnostic for cancer and has many limitations.

CBC And Blood Chemistry

CBC and blood chemistry tests are considered the beginning point in cancer screening. These tests give baseline values and are extremely helpful in finding the cause of certain disease patterns. Again, these tests are used as tools and are not the final word in the diagnosing of cancer. More sophisticated CBC analysis is accomplished by Carbon Based Corporation.

Colonoscopy

Colonoscopy is a procedure that allows the entire colon to be visualized. During this procedure, a biopsy of normal and/or diseased tissue is accomplished. Colonoscopy usually takes about forty-five minutes to perform, and the patient is given a general anesthetic. It is an outpatient procedure. Colonoscopy is a screening test for cancers of the large bowel. For individu-als with increased risk of bowel cancer, it is recommended that this procedure be performed every three years.

CT Scan

Computed Tomography (CT Scan) is valuable in detecting cancer in surrounding tissue and organs. However, some types of cancer may not always show up on this form of imaging. It may be necessary to have more sophisticated imaging, such as Magnetic Resonance Imaging (MRI) and bone scan. CT scans are also used to monitor an individual's response to therapeutic treatment. During the procedure, the patient lies very still on a table. The table passes through the X-ray machine, which is shaped like a doughnut with a large hole. The machine, which is linked to a computer, rotates around the patient, taking pictures of one thin slice of tissue after another. To obtain a clearer picture, the patient may be given a solution of contrast material to drink or get an injection into an arm vein before the CT is done. The length of the procedure depends on the size of the area to be X-rayed. The CT scan is relatively painless. Some mild heat may be experienced if contrast material is used. If you are allergic to certain types of contrast material, notify your physician or technician before beginning the process.

Darkfield Microscopy

This type of testing views tiny particles in the blood and blood components. Motion study and cell characteristics are noted in detail with Darkfield technology. Darkfield is used to study live blood, magnified about 1,500X, and projects it onto a video screen. A physician skilled in the use of this type of testing can pick up on early signs of illness and design appropriate treatment. Darkfield microscopy is not diagnostic for cancer and also has limitations. It is a useful as an adjunct form of analysis to design a better treatment regimen in cancer treatment.

ELISA/ACT

ELISA/ACT is a test that was developed in 1984 for the purpose of evaluation of delayed immune response and immune reactivity to certain offending agents. To begin the repair process of the immune system, offending agents need to be identified and avoided. These substances may facilitate further cancer development. This test can help identify and assist the clinician in developing a more effective treatment strategy. Contact *ELISA/ACT Lab at 1.800.553.5472* for information on this type of testing. This is not a diagnostic test for cancer.

Genetic Testing

Developments in gene testing are phenomenal. Gene testing examines blood, other body fluids, or tissue for biochemical, chromosomal, or genetic markers for some anomaly that flags a disease or disorder. Gene causation for cancer is an area of continued exploration among cancer researchers. Some inherited forms of cancers are now linked to specific genes. Some of these genes have been located and can be tested:

- adenocarcinoma of lung, pancreas, and colon- K-ras

- brain cancer—MSH2, MLH1, PMS1, PMS2

- breast cancer—BRCA1, cyclin D1, erb-B2

- colon and uterine cancer—BRCA2, DCC, K-ras, APC

- endocrine cancer—MEN1, MEN2a

- leukemia—ATM, BLM, FA-A,C

- lung cancer—myc, erb-B2, cyclin D1, abl

- lymphoma—ATM, BLM

- pancreatic cancer—p16, BRCA2, MLH1, MSH2, PMS1, PMS2, K-ras

- skin cancer—p16 (melanoma), BLM

- thyroid cancer—MEN2B

Heavy Metal Analysis

Continuous heavy metal toxicity leads to both immune and metabolic suppression. A hair analysis test for heavy metal toxicity is a good tool to use since the hair provides a record of these toxic substances. This test is inexpensive, non-invasive, and easy to perform. A twenty-four-hour urine analysis is also useful in detecting heavy metal toxicity, as is a blood analysis.

ELISA/ACT is also used to determine, more accurately, tissue levels of heavy metals, because the measurements are accomplished on white blood cells. Chelation therapy (oral and intravenous) is available to detoxify the body tissue. In addition, biological dentistry is also a type of therapy that assists in the removal of mercury and nickel fillings that are known to cause toxicity.

Stool Testing for Blood (Hemoccult)

This test is the first line in detecting rectal bleeding that may be associated with colon cancer. This screening test should be given every time you have a major physical exam.

Individualized Optimal Nutrition (ION)

ION is a useful test that focuses upon prevention and nutrition. The ION Program is broken down into five profiles that cover specific testing areas. The following briefly describes each of the five profiles.

> **Amino acids:** Amino acids are the substances of which protein is made. When you eat a protein food, digestive enzymes break it down into amino acids to use for some vital work: brain function, immune system, repair of tissues, energy generation, and blood sugar regulation. Inadequate diets, stress, and poor digestion can deplete amino acids in your body, adversely affecting these functions. It is most often

noticed as fatigue. This profile measures amino acid deficiencies in your system.

Vitamins and minerals: B-vitamins and nutrient minerals are not stored in the body, so we must eat them in our diet. They are essential for converting food into usable energy for many vital functions: nerve transmission, digestion, antibody production, and growth and repair of tissue. For this reason, deficiencies have been associated with heart disease, cancer, and a host of other degenerative processes. In many cases, dietary sources provide inadequate amounts. This profile measures your adequacy of these important nutrients through both organic acids and minerals.

Antioxidants: Normal biological processes and environmental pollutants produce unstable molecules called free radicals that wreak havoc on tissues by setting tiny "fires" of oxidation. This oxidative stress is continual and requires antioxidants, indispensable molecular "fire-extinguishers," to shield against excessive free radical damage. Poor antioxidant protection has been associated with every major disease. This profile measures your free radical activity and levels of antioxidant vitamins.

Regulation of inflammatory processes: Fat is necessary for health. Nerve coverings and all cell membranes are made of fatty acids. They produce hormone-like substances that regulate inflammation. They protect against heart disease and cancer and help our skin, hair, and joints stay young and supple. Most of us have diets rich in "bad" fats, hydrogenated and trans fats, common in processed foods. We need more of the "good" fats from fish, flaxseed, and vegetable/nut oils. This profile determines your critical fatty acid balance.

Screening for organ system disease risk: Like gauges in a car, certain chemicals in your body warn of potential problems, so that you can make corrections before things get out of hand. This profile uses traditional and newer measures of blood chemicals to detect overt disease or risk of developing health problems. It screens for diabetes, liver disorders, kidney problems, thyroid function, and heart disease risk and can be a very effective prevention screen for cancer.

The comprehensive report that is produced for the ION test is a bound booklet containing five sections of information. Section one is a series of graphs showing overall scores in key nutrient-related areas. Section two is a table of recommended supplementation levels, where each nutrient is evaluated from the test results. Vitamins, minerals, fatty acids, amino acids, and other special nutrients are covered. The remaining sections provide increasing levels of detail about your specific test results, including paragraphs discussing each abnormality, pages of laboratory reports, and a glossary of terms so you can look up meanings of the scientific terms. By applying the ION program to your life, you can take a positive step in assuring that your body has a daily supply of the high quality nutrients it needs to function best. If you change nothing else in your lifestyle, you have still given yourself an edge toward your personal best level of health and energy. *Contact MetaMetrix, Inc. at 1.800.221.4640* for more information.

Mammography, Ultrasound, and Biopsy

A screening mammogram is an X-ray of the breast, used to detect breast changes in women who have no signs of breast cancer. It usually involves two X-rays of each breast. Using a mammogram, it is possible to detect a tumor that cannot be felt. This is a routine form of testing for women over the age of thirty-five that have a high risk for breast cancer. For prevention of breast cancer, a mammogram is recommended for women over age forty, coupled with a breast self-exam at least one time monthly. Confirmatory ultrasound is a valuable form of imaging that is noninvasive. This should be utilized if mammography is unclear. Biopsy should be performed if the lesion is not clearly distinguished. If there is any suspicion at all, all three diagnostic tools should be utilized along with tumor markers, hormone receptor assay, and confirmatory CT and/or MRI.

MRI

Magnetic Resonance Imaging (MRI) is a sophisticated form of imaging that is even more powerful than the CT scan. In the detection of cancer that affects soft tissue, the MRI is superior to the CT scan. Contrast material can be administered to enhance the visibility of abnormal tissue. For individuals that have a fear of closed places, there are MRI units that are open. MRI is relatively painless. If contrast material is given, there may be some mild heat sensation felt because of the contrast material. If you are allergic to certain types of contrast material, notify your physician or technician ahead of time.

Oxidative Protection Panel

An Oxidative Protection Panel includes a serum lipid peroxide level. Lipid peroxides are the products of the chemical damage done by oxygen free radicals to the lipid components of cell membranes. This oxidative damage caused by free radical pathology is thought to be a basic mechanism underlying many diverse pathological conditions—atherosclerosis, cancer, aging, rheumatic diseases, allergic inflammation, cardiac and cerebral ischemia, respiratory distress syndrome, various liver disorders, irradiation and thermal injury, and toxicity induced by certain metals, solvents, pesticides, and drugs. A serum lipid peroxide level, therefore, measures the overall potential for oxygen free radical pathology, the risk for degenerative processes, and the need for compensatory antioxidant supplementation. High serum lipid peroxide levels indicate excessive oxygen free radical lipid peroxidation.

Mechanism underlying pathology: This fundamental process underlying pathological conditions demonstrates the widespread application of this concept to many different diseases, including cancer. Chemically, a substance is oxidized when electrons are removed and reduced when electrons are added. All chemical reactions involve the transfer of electrons. The body generates energy by gradually oxidizing its food in a controlled fashion and storing it in the form of chemical potential energy called ATP. This oxidation process removes electrons sequentially in a kind of bucket brigade, passing the electrons to their final recipient, molecular oxygen, forming water and generating ATP. Ironically, this energy generation mechanism that is so essential to life can also set the stage for cell damage.

The oxidation of foodstuffs is like a controlled fire that liberates energy but can also let sparks fly, giving rise to potential damage. The sparks in this analogy are free electrons escaping the transport system or electrons freed by lack of chain-terminating oxygen (hypoxic conditions). These unpaired electrons readily form free radical molecules that are highly unstable and chemically reactive. It is these free radical molecules, which rapidly react with other molecules, setting off a chain reaction of radical formation similar to an atomic explosion. The unsaturated lipid molecules of cell membranes are particularly susceptible to this damaging reaction process and readily contribute to the uncontrolled chain reaction. However, other biological molecules are also susceptible to damage, including protein enzymes, DNA, and RNA.

Hence, in one process, all levels of cell function may be disrupted. This is why free radical pathology is thought to be such a basic mechanism of tissue injury and end-stage pathology. It is also clear that environmental agents may initiate free radical problems. The toxicity of lead, cadmium, pesticides, ionizing radiation, cigarette smoke, and alcohol may all be due to their free radical initiating ability. Cancer can be initiated by free radical formation, and it is essential to remove the exposure and strengthen the defense and resistance to these offending agents.

Role of antioxidants: Later in the book I discuss the role of specific antioxidants and their usage in cancer. However, briefly, antioxidants prevent the free radical chain propagation effect; the body uses antioxidants (chemical electron sinks) that quench the biochemical fire. The antioxidants include enzymes such as glutathione peroxidase, superoxide dismutase, and catalase. Vitamins A, C, and E, beta carotene, and coenzyme Q10 are potent antioxidants, which may be their principle role in the body. All these compounds help to control the propagation of free radical pathology in the tissues.

A measure of total serum lipid peroxidation has proven to be a simple, inexpensive, and accurate means of reflecting whole-body free radical activity. This test is presently gaining general acceptance in the research laboratory as a simple, standard means of assessing the body's antioxidant capability or overall oxidative stress. *Contact MetaMetrix, Inc. at 1.800.221.4640* for more information.

113

Pap Smear

The traditional Pap smear was introduced about fifty years ago by Dr. George Papanicolaou. This test was designed for the purpose of the detection of cervical cancer. The accuracy of this screening test depends upon the technician's skill in reading the sample. There are many false negatives in traditional Pap smears. There are other methods that are more accurate. One system is called Accuslide®. Accuslide® use the latest technology for cancer screening of the cervix. Most laboratories are current on the latest tissue screening techniques.

Diagnostic Testing Specific for Prostate Cancer

Prostate, PSA, and ultrasound: Prostate cancer is the second leading cause of cancer-related deaths among American men. Prostate-specific antigen (PSA) is a blood antigen that is found to be elevated in cases of prostate cancer, prostate enlargement, and prostate inflammation. If cancer of the prostate is suspected, then the PSA blood testing must be accompanied by prostate ultrasound and biopsy. Adjunct testing, like AMAS, could give a better assessment. Elevated PSA does not always indicate the presence of cancer. The false positive rate for PSA can be as high as 70%. Establishing a baseline is important. A good place to start is as follows:

- PSA level

- free PSA level

- RT-PCR PSA if indicated

- prostates acid phosphatase test

- Gleason score

- other tests and imaging (CEA, CGA, NSE, testosterone assay, SHBG, MRI, US, etc.), if necessary

Some other tests and imaging worthy of consideration include:

RT-PCR PSA: This test does not measure the amount of protein in the blood. It identifies prostate cancer cells in the blood, using molecular staging. These PSA-secreting cells are not seen in healthy men. However, they are expected in the blood of men with non-organ-confined prostate cancer. This technique is seldom used because of variations of results. With more consistent use, this form of testing is more sensitive and specific because it is measuring on the molecular level. This form of blood testing detects PSA signs in pelvic lymph nodes with more sensitivity than other traditional blood tests. Patients can use this form of testing to establish a baseline and for therapeutic monitoring.

Endorectal MRI: This imaging technique utilizes a long narrow tube that contains radio-frequency coils. This tube is inserted into the rectum while the MRI scan is formed. It gives a clearer picture of the prostate gland and surrounding tissues. It improves the ability to measure the size of the cancer. It detects the cancer more accurately.

MRI: MRI is the method of choice for detecting whether prostate cancer has spread. It is a more specific form of imaging, and it can detect soft tissue metastasis very well.

CT Scan: CT scans have not demonstrated favorable results in detecting soft tissue cancers. It is not considered the best choice of imaging for the prostate.

Power Doppler Angiography: This form of imaging is effective in looking at blood vessels and is able to detect blood flow to the prostate. It is able to pick up cancers that are also readily detected by digital rectal exam and MRI tests. The Power Doppler is an effective method of detecting early prostate cancer and it is cost-effective. For further information on prostate cancer herbal therapy, go to the herbal therapy section entitled PC SPES and read the prostate cancer case study toward the end of the book. For further information, consult:

1. *The Best Options for Diagnosing and Treating Prostate Cancer by* James Lewis Jr., Ph.D. ISBN 1-883257-042

2. *The Herbal Remedy for Prostate Cancer* by James Lewis Jr., Ph.D. ISBN 1-883257-02-6

Tumor Markers

Tumor markers are used to detect and monitor therapy. There are different categories, and you should ask your physician for specific details regarding these markers. Some markers are tumor-specific, tumor-associated antigens, hormones, and/or enzymes. When there is any suspicion of cancer, a tumor marker assay can be utilized and is advised. Some common tumor-specific markers are AFP, CEA, CA125, CA15-3, CA19-9, and CA27.29. These tests should be utilized as part of the diagnosis and treatment of cancer. Consult your physician for further information.

Early Detection Test Summary

The following table is a summary of the American Cancer Society recommendations for the early detection of cancer in people without symptoms.

Table 1.0

Summary of American Cancer Society Recommendations for the Early Detection of Cancer in Asymptomatic People Test Sex Age Frequency

Test	Sex	Age and Frequency
Sigmoidoscopy, preferably flexible	M/F	50 and over; Every 3–5 years
Fecal Occult Blood Test	M/F	50 and over; Every year
Digital Rectal Exam	M/F	40 and over; Every year
Prostate Exam*	M	50 and over; Every year
Pap Test	F	All women who are or have been sexually active, or who have reached age 18, should have annual Pap test and pelvic examination. After a woman has had three or more consecutive and satisfactory Pap tests, annual Pap tests may be performed less frequently at the discretion of her physician.
Breast Self-examination	F	20 and over; Every month
Breast Clinical Examination	F	20–40 Every 1–2 years Over 40 Every year
Mammography**	F	40–49 Every 1–2 years 50 and over Every year

*Annual digital rectal examination and prostate-specific antigen should be performed on men 50 years and older. If either result is abnormal, further evaluation should be considered.

**Screening mammography should begin by age 40.

- -

Chapter 7

Conventional Cancer Treatment

Both conventional and alternative medical treatments have much to offer in cancer therapy. As the science of medicine and integrative treatment strategies advance, these new developments must be clearly explained to the individual considering the treatment.

In conventional treatment, it is common to use chemotherapy, surgery, radiation, and biological therapy. These therapies may be used in combination, depending upon the type of cancer. In this section, we will briefly discuss chemotherapy and radiotherapy, which is also called radiation therapy.

CHEMOTHERAPY

There are many forms of chemotherapy with varied results. Not all regimens are the same. It is always prudent to implement integrative treatment to combat the negative effects of chemotherapy. You may not be settled with chemotherapy or you may be unsure as to whether it is right for you. This is why it is vital to research and get the expert advice from your oncologist and alternative health care physician before making a decision.

Chemotherapeutic agents have different classifications and actions:

- alkylating agents and platinum agents
- antimetabolites
- anti-tumor compounds
- anti-tumor antibiotics
- biological response modifiers
- hormones and anti-hormone agents
- microtubule inhibiting agents
- chromatin function inhibitors
- Molecular Targeted Agents

In Appendix 1, you will find a table of classifications with common and trade names. In Appendix 6, you will also find a sample natural medicine, oral treatment regimen that can minimize the negative effects and adverse reactions encountered by the use of these agents. Please be advised that it is essential that you remain under the care of your health care team for the best treatment options. Your team must include a specialist in natural medicine.

Molecular Targeted Agents

Gleevec: Gleevec is used in the treatment of chronic myeloid leukemia (CML). It is the first approved "molecularly targeted" drug. This drug targets the gene defect found in cells of patients with this type of cancer. Gleevec in the treatment of CML has been miraculous. From a study, results were reported in *The New England Journal of Medicine*, April 2001 issue that fifty-three out of fifty-four human subjects had restored normal blood values. This is excellent news! Gleevec is being studied in other cancers including lung and gastrointestinal cancers.

Herceptin: Herceptin is a monoclonal antibody that seeks out a specific target antigen known as HER2 receptors that lie on the surface of certain cancer cells. Women with breast cancer should be tested for the HER2 receptor site. Some women may express multiple copies of the gene that produces a protein HER2 growth factor, which plays a role proliferation of cancer cells. In women that express HER2 protein, Herceptin binds to the cell and helps shrink the tumor. Herceptin has fewer side effects than traditional chemotherapy agents. The most common adverse reaction is fever and chills and usually not severe. Herceptin may cause damage to heart tissue and should be discontinued immediately if this has occurred.

Rituxan: This agent is used in B-cell type non-Hodgkin's lymphoma (NHL), targeting a certain antigen known as CD-20. Rituxan is a monoclonal antibody that binds to CD-20 and destroys the cell. Currently, its response efficacy is between 40–50%. This agent does have some side effects associated with it that are usually mild, including fever, chills, rash, and nausea. There have been some cases of life-threatening respiratory adverse events that are associated with allergy to the agent.

How Does Chemotherapy Work?

Normal cells grow and die in a controlled way. When cancer occurs, cells in the body that are not normal keep dividing and forming more cells without control. Anticancer drugs destroy cancer cells by stopping them from growing or multiplying. Healthy cells can also be harmed, especially those that divide quickly. Harm to healthy cells is what causes side effects. These cells usually repair themselves after chemotherapy.

What Can Chemotherapy Do?

Depending on the type of cancer and how advanced it is, chemotherapy can be used for different goals:

- To remit the cancer. Cancer is considered in remission when the patient remains free of evidence of cancer cells.

- To control the cancer. This is done by keeping the cancer from spreading, slowing the cancer's growth, and killing cancer cells that may have spread to other parts of the body from the original tumor.

- To relieve symptoms that the cancer may cause. Relieving symptoms, such as pain, can help patients live more comfortably.

Is Chemotherapy Used with Other Treatments?

Sometimes chemotherapy is the only treatment a patient receives. More often, however, chemotherapy is used in addition to surgery and/or biological therapy to:

- Shrink a tumor before surgery or radiation therapy. This is called neo-adjuvant therapy.

- Help destroy any cancer cells that may remain after surgery and/or radiation therapy. This is called adjuvant chemotherapy.

- Make radiation therapy and biological therapy work better.

- Help destroy cancer if it recurs or has spread to other parts of the body from the original tumor.

Which Drugs Are Given?

Some chemotherapy drugs are used for many different types of cancer, while others might be used for just one or two types of cancer. Regardless, staying informed about your chemotherapy regimen is very important in order to know the effectiveness of the regimen and possible side reactions or potential hazards of the therapy. See Appendix 1 for a general list of the common chemotherapeutic agents.

Your doctor recommends a treatment plan based on:

- what kind of cancer you have
- what part of the body the cancer is found in
- the effect of cancer on your normal body functions
- your general health

What about Clinical Trials?

Clinical trials test many types of treatments, such as new drugs, new approaches to surgery or radiation therapy, new combinations of treatments, or new methods such as gene therapy. The goal of this research is to find better ways to treat cancer and help cancer patients. There are different types of clinical trials: Phase I, Phase II, and Phase III trials. Each is one of the final stages of a long and careful cancer research process. If your doctor does not suggest you take part in a clinical trial, you may want to ask about clinical trials as a treatment choice for you.

Possible benefits of clinical trials:

- Clinical trials offer high-quality cancer care
- If a new treatment approach is proven to work and you are taking it, you may be among the first to benefit
- By looking at the pros and cons of clinical trials and other treatment choices, you are taking an active role in a decision that affects your life
- You have the chance to help others and improve cancer treatment

Possible drawbacks:

- New treatments under study are not always better than, or even as good as, standard treatment.

- Even if a new treatment has benefits, it may not work for you.

- In a study, if you are randomly assigned to have standard treatment instead of the new treatment being tested, it may not be as effective as the new approach.

- Health insurance and managed care providers do not always cover all patient care costs in a study.

- Before deciding to join a clinical trial, you will want to ask important questions such as: What are the possible short- and long-term risks, side effects, and benefits to me? How could the study affect my daily life? Will I have to pay for any treatment, tests, or other charges?

Ask Your Doctor About Chemotherapy

- Why do I need chemotherapy?

- What are the benefits of chemotherapy?

- What are the risks of chemotherapy?

- Are there any other possible treatment methods for my type of cancer?

- What is the standard care for my type of cancer?

- Are there any clinical trials for my type of cancer?

About your treatment:

- How many treatments will I be given?

- What drug or drugs will I be taking?

- How will the drugs be given?

- Where will I get my treatment?

- How long will each treatment last?

About side effects:

- What are the possible side effects of the chemotherapy?

- When are side effects likely to occur?

- What side effects are more likely to be related to my type of cancer?

- Are there any side effects that I should report right away?

- What can I do to relieve the side effects?

About contacting medical staff:

- How do I contact a health professional after hours, and when should I call?

Hints for Talking with Your Doctor

These tips might help you keep track of the information you learn during visits with your doctor.

- Bring a friend or family member to sit with you while you talk with your doctor. This person can help you understand what your doctor says during your visit and help refresh your memory afterward.

- Ask your doctor for printed information that is available on your cancer and treatment.

- You or the person who goes with you may want to take notes during your appointment.

- Ask your doctor to slow down when you need more time to write.

- You may want to ask if you can use a tape recorder during your visit. Take notes from the tape after the visit is finished. That way, you can review your conversation later as many times as you wish.

How Often and for How Long Will I Get Chemotherapy?

How often and how long you get chemotherapy depends on:

- the kind of cancer you have

- the goals of the treatment

- the drugs that are used

- how your body responds to them

You may get treatment every day, every week, or every month. Chemotherapy is often given in cycles that include treatment periods alternated with rest periods. Rest periods give your body a chance to build healthy new cells and regain its strength. Ask your health care provider to tell you how long and how often you may expect to get treatment. Sticking with your treatment schedule is very important for the drugs to work right. Schedules may need to be changed for holidays and other reasons. If you miss a treatment session or skip a dose of the drug, contact your doctor. Sometimes, your doctor may need to delay a treatment based on the results of certain blood tests. Your doctor will let you know what to do during this time and when to start your treatment again.

How Is Chemotherapy Given?

Chemotherapy can be given in several different ways: intravenously (through a vein), by mouth, through an injection, through use of a port or pump, or applied on the skin.

> **By vein (intravenous, or IV, treatment):** Chemotherapy is most often given intravenously (IV) through a vein. Usually, a thin needle is inserted into a vein on the hand or lower arm at the beginning of each treatment session and is removed at the end of the ses-

sion. If you feel coolness, burning, or other unusual sensation in the area of the needle stick when the IV is started, tell your doctor or nurse. Also report any pain, burning, skin redness, swelling, or discomfort that occurs during or after an IV treatment.

Chemotherapy can also be delivered by IV through catheters, ports, and pumps. A catheter is a soft, thin, flexible tube that is placed in a large vein in the body and remains there as long as it is needed. Patients who need to have many IV treatments often have a catheter, so a needle does not have to be used each time. Drugs can be given and blood samples can be drawn through this catheter.

IV port: Sometimes, the catheter is attached to a small, round, plastic or metal disc, placed under the skin and attached to the vein. The port is surgically placed and is advised if there are several rounds of treatment recommended. This can prevent vein injury induced by repeated use of chemo agents. The port can be used for as long as it is needed. These ports after repeated use can become clogged and worn and may need to replaced. It is essential that the ports be carefully flushed with heparin and saline to preserve its use and function.

Pump: A pump, which is used to control how fast the drug goes into a catheter or port, is sometimes used. There are two types of pumps. An external pump remains outside the body. Most are portable; they allow a person to move around while the pump is being used. An internal pump is placed inside the body during surgery, usually right under the skin. Pumps contain a small storage area for the drug and allow people to go about their normal activities. Catheters, ports, and pumps cause no pain if they are properly placed and cared for, although a person is aware they are there.

By mouth (orally): The drug is given in pill, capsule, or liquid form. You swallow the drug, just as you do many other medicines.

By injection: A needle and syringe are used to give the drug in one of several ways:

- intra-muscular, or IM (into a muscle)

- subcutaneous, or SQ or SC (under the skin)

- intra-lesion, or IL (directly into a cancerous area in the skin)

Topically: The drug is applied on the surface of the skin.

How Will I Feel During Chemotherapy?

Most people receiving chemotherapy find that they tire easily, but many feel well enough to continue to lead active lives. Each person and treatment is different, so it is not always possible to tell exactly how you will react. Your general state of health, the type and extent of cancer you have, and the kind of drugs you are receiving can all affect how well you feel. You may want to have someone available to drive you to and from treatment if, for example, you are taking medicine for nausea or vomiting that could make you tired. You may also feel especially tired from the chemotherapy as early as one day after a treatment and for several days afterwards. It may help to schedule your treatment when you can take off work the day of and the day after your treatment. If you have young children, you may want to schedule the treatment when you have someone to help at home the day of and at least the day after your treatment. Ask your doctor when your greatest fatigue or other side effects are likely to occur.

Most people can continue working while receiving chemotherapy. However, you may need to change your work schedule for a while if your chemotherapy makes you feel very tired or have other side effects. Talk with your employer about your needs and wishes. You may be able to agree on a part-time schedule, find an area for a short nap during the day, or perhaps you can do some of your work at home. Under federal and state laws, some employers may be required to let you work a flexible schedule to meet your treatment needs. To find out about your on-the-job protections, check with a social worker or your congressional or state representative.

Can I take other medicines while I am getting chemotherapy? Some medicines may interfere or react with the effects of your chemotherapy. Give your doctor a list of all the medicines you take before you start treatment. Include:

- the name of each drug

- the dosage

- the reason you take it

- how often you take it

How will I know if my chemotherapy is working? Your doctor and nurse will use several ways to see how well your treatments are working. You may have physical exams and tests often. Always feel free to ask your doctor about the test results and what they show about your progress. Tests and exams can tell a lot about how chemotherapy is working; however, side effects tell very little. Sometimes, people think that if they have no side effects, the drugs are not working; or if they do have side effects, the drugs are working well. But side effects vary so much from person to person and from drug to drug that they are not a sign of whether the treatment is working or not.

Side Effects Encountered During Chemotherapy

Because cancer cells may grow and divide more rapidly than normal cells, many anticancer drugs are made to kill growing cells. But certain normal, healthy cells also multiply quickly, and chemotherapy can affect these cells too. This damage to normal cells causes side effects. The fast-growing, normal cells most likely to be affected are blood cells forming in the bone and cells in the digestive tract (mouth, stomach, intestines, and esophagus), reproductive system (sexual organs), and hair follicles. Some anticancer drugs may affect cells of vital organs, such as the heart, kidney, bladder, lungs, and nervous system. You may have none of these side effects or just a few. The kinds of side effects you have, and how severe they are, depend on the type and dose of chemotherapy you get and how your body reacts to it. Before starting chemotherapy, your doctor will discuss the side effects that you are most likely to get with the drugs you will be receiving. Before starting the treatment, you will be asked to sign a consent form. You should be given all the facts about treatment, including the drugs you will be given and their side effects, before you sign the consent form.

> **How long do side effects last?** Normal cells usually recover when chemotherapy is over, so most side effects gradually go away after treatment ends and the healthy cells have a chance to grow normally. The time it takes to get over side effects depends on many things, including your overall health and the kind of chemotherapy you have been taking. On some occasions, chemotherapy can cause permanent changes or damage to the heart, lungs, nerves, kidneys, reproductive, or other organs. And certain types of chemotherapy may have delayed effects, such as a second cancer that shows up many years later. Ask your doctor about the chances of any serious, long-term effects that can result from the treatment you are receiving (but remember to balance

your concerns with the immediate threat of your cancer).

Great progress has been made in preventing and treating some of chemotherapy's common, as well as rare, serious side effects. Many new drugs and treatment methods destroy cancer more effectively while doing less harm to the body's healthy cells. The side effects of chemotherapy can be unpleasant, but they must be measured against the treatment's ability to destroy cancer. Medicines can help prevent some side effects, such as nausea. Sometimes, people receiving chemotherapy become discouraged about the length of time their treatment is taking or the side effects they are having. If that happens to you, talk to your doctor or nurse. They may be able to suggest ways to make side effects easier to deal with or reduce them.

It is essential to consider integrating your therapy with proper nutritional replacement. In many cases, the body is deprived of vital nutrients and minerals that the chemotherapy depletes. IV nutritional replacement is recommended. Some of the common side effects can improve, if not be abated, by nutritional support therapy.

Below, you will find suggestions for managing some of the more common of chemotherapy.

Fatigue: Fatigue, feeling tired, and lacking energy is the most common symptom reported by cancer patients. The exact cause is not always known. It can be due to your disease, chemotherapy, radiation, surgery, low blood counts, lack of sleep, pain, stress, or poor appetite, along with many other factors. Fatigue from cancer feels different from fatigue of everyday life.

Fatigue caused by chemotherapy can appear suddenly. Patients with cancer have described it as a total lack of energy and have used words such as "worn out," "drained," and "wiped out" to describe their fatigue. And rest does not always relieve it. Not everyone feels the same kind of fatigue. You may not feel tired, while someone else does, or your fatigue may not last as long as someone else's does. It can last days, weeks, or months. But severe fatigue does go away gradually as the tumor responds to treatment.

How can I cope with fatigue?

- Plan your day so that you have time to rest.

- Take short naps or breaks, rather than one long rest period.

- Save your energy for the most important things.

- Try easier or shorter versions of activities you enjoy.

- Take short walks or do light exercise if possible. You may find this helps with fatigue.

- Talk to your health care provider about ways to save your energy and treat your fatigue.

- Eat as well as you can and drink plenty of fluids. Eat small amounts at a time if it is helpful.

- Join a support group. Sharing your feelings with others can ease the burden of fatigue. You can learn how others deal with their fatigue. Your health care provider can put you in touch with a support group in your area.

- Limit the amount of caffeine and alcohol you drink.

- Allow others to do some things for you that you usually do.

- Keep a diary of how you feel each day. This will help you plan your daily activities.

- Report any changes in energy level to your doctor or nurse.

Nausea and vomiting: Many patients fear that they will have nausea and vomiting while receiving chemotherapy. But new drugs have made these side effects far less common and, when they do occur, much less severe. Anti-nausea drugs can prevent or lessen nausea and vomiting in most patients. Different drugs work for different people, and you may need more than one drug to get relief. Do not give up. Continue to work with your doctor and nurse to find the drug or drugs that work best for you. Also, be sure to tell your doctor or nurse if you are very nauseated or have vomited for more than a day, or if your vomiting is so bad that you cannot keep liquids down.

What can I do if I have nausea and vomiting?

- Drink liquids at least an hour before or after mealtime, instead of with your meals. Drink frequently and drink small amounts.

- Eat and drink slowly.

- Eat small meals throughout the day, instead of one, two, or three large meals.

- Eat foods cold or at room temperature so you won't be bothered by strong smells.

- Chew your food well for easier digestion.

- If nausea is a problem in the morning, try eating dry foods like cereal, toast, or crackers before getting up. (Do not try this if you have mouth or throat sores or are troubled by a lack of saliva.)

- Drink cool, clear, unsweetened fruit juices, such as apple or grape juice (or light-colored sodas, such as ginger ale, that have lost their fizz and do not have caffeine).

- Suck on mints or tart candies. (Do not use tart candies if you have mouth or throat sores.)

- Prepare and freeze meals in advance for days when you do not feel like cooking.

- Wear loose-fitting clothes.

- Breathe deeply and slowly when you feel nauseated.

- Distract yourself by chatting with friends or family members, listening to music, or watching a movie or TV show.

- Use relaxation techniques.

- Try to avoid odors that bother you, such as cooking smells, smoke, or perfume.

- Avoid sweet, fried, or fatty foods.

- Rest, but do not lie flat for at least two hours after you finish a meal.

- Avoid eating for at least a few hours before treatment if nausea usually occurs during chemotherapy.

- Eat a light meal before treatment.

Pain: Chemotherapy drugs can cause some side effects that are painful. The drugs can damage nerves, leading to burning, numbness, tingling, or shooting pain, most often in the fingers or toes. Some drugs can also cause mouth sores, headaches, muscle pains, and stomach pains. Not everyone with cancer or who receives chemotherapy experiences pain from the disease or its treatment. But if you do, it can be relieved. The first step to take is to talk with your doctor, nurse, and pharmacist about your pain. They need to know as many details about your pain as possible. You may want to describe your pain to your family and friends. They can help you talk to your caregivers about your pain, especially if you are too tired or in too much pain to talk to them yourself.

You need to tell your doctor, nurse, pharmacist, and family, or friends:

- where you feel pain

- what it feels like—sharp, dull, throbbing, steady

- how strong the pain feels

- how long it lasts

- what eases the pain; what makes the pain worse

- what medicines you are taking for the pain, and how much relief you get from them

Using a pain scale is helpful in describing how much pain you are feeling. Try to assign a number from 0 to 10 to your pain level. If you have no pain, use a 0. As the numbers get higher, they stand for pain that is getting worse. A 10 means the pain is as bad as it can be. You may wish to use your own pain scale, using numbers from 0 to 5 or even 0 to 100. Be sure to let others know what pain scale you are using, and use the same scale each time. For example, "My pain is 7 on a scale of 0 to 10." The goal of pain control is to prevent pain that can be prevented and treat the pain that can't. To do this, try these suggestions:

- If you have persistent or chronic pain, take your pain medicine on a regular schedule (by the clock).

- Do not skip doses of your scheduled pain medicine. If you wait to take pain medicine until you feel pain, it is harder to control.

- Try using relaxation exercises at the same time you take medicine for the pain. This may help to lessen tension, reduce anxiety, and manage pain.

Some people with chronic or persistent pain that is usually controlled by medicine can have breakthrough pain. This occurs when moderate to severe pain "breaks through" or is felt for a short time. If you experience this pain, use a short-acting medicine ordered by your doctor. Don't wait for the pain to get worse. If you do, it may be harder to control. There are many different medicines and methods available to control cancer pain. You should expect your doctor to seek all the information and resources necessary to make you as comfortable as possible. If you are in pain and your doctor has no further suggestions, ask to see a pain specialist or have your doctor consult with a pain specialist. A pain specialist may be an oncologist, anesthesiologist, neurologist, neurosurgeon, other doctor, nurse, or pharmacist.

Hair loss: Hair loss is a common side effect of chemotherapy, but not all drugs cause hair loss. Your doctor can tell you if hair loss might occur with the drug or drugs you are taking. When hair loss does occur, the hair may become thinner or fall out entirely. Hair loss can occur on all parts of the body, including the head, face, arms and legs, underarms, and pubic area. The hair usually grows back after the treatments are over. Some people even start to get their hair back while they are still having treatments. Sometimes, hair may grow back a different color or texture. Hair loss does not always happen right away. It may begin several weeks after the first treatment or after a few treatments. Many people say their head becomes sensitive before losing hair. Hair may fall out gradually or in clumps. Any hair that is still growing may become dull and dry.

How can I care for my scalp and hair during chemotherapy?

- Use a mild shampoo.

- Use a soft hairbrush.

- Use low heat when drying your hair.

- Have your hair cut short. A shorter style will make your hair look thicker and fuller. It also will make hair loss easier to manage if it occurs.

- Use a sunscreen, sun block, hat, or scarf to protect your scalp from the sun if you lose hair on your head.

- Avoid brush rollers to set your hair.

- Avoid dying, perming, or relaxing your hair.

Some people who lose all or most of their hair choose to wear turbans, scarves, caps, wigs, or hairpieces. Others leave their head uncovered. Still others switch back and forth, depending on whether they are in public or at home with friends and family members. There are no "right" or "wrong" choices; do whatever feels comfortable for you.

If you choose to cover your head:

- Get your wig or hairpiece before you lose a lot of hair. That way, you can match your current hairstyle and color. You may be able to buy a wig or hairpiece at a specialty shop just for cancer patients. Someone may even come to your home to help you. You also can buy a wig or hairpiece through a catalog or by phone.

- You may also consider borrowing a wig or hairpiece, rather than buying one. Check with the nurse or social work department at your hospital about resources for free wigs in your community.

- Take your wig to your hairdresser or the shop where it was purchased for styling and cutting to frame your face.

- Some health insurance policies cover the cost of a hairpiece needed because of cancer treatment. It is also a tax-deductible expense. Be sure to check your policy and ask your doctor for a "prescription." Losing hair from your head, face, or body can be hard to accept.

- Feeling angry or depressed is common. At the same time, keep in mind that it is a temporary side effect. Talking about your feelings can help. If possible, share your thoughts with someone who has had a similar experience.

Drug-induced hair loss, particularly involving chemotherapeutic agents, is a common adverse effect. Some of the drugs that can cause hair loss are Gentamyacin, Coumadin, Prozac Dilantin, ACE inhibitors, betablockers, Adriamycin, Vincristine, Bromocriptine, Naprosen, Tagamet, Zantac, and Ibuprofen.

Hair loss associated with low thyroid function is another common occurrence, especially when receiving chemotherapy. It is essential that the thyroid be monitored during treatment. Monitoring TSH, T4, and Free T3 reference values to be sure that they are within normal functional limits is essential and your physician should be aware of this important detail.

Hair loss associated with nutritional deficiency is also common in cancer treatment. This is why it is vitally important to replace nutrients intravenously after receiving conventional treatment. In *Appendixes 3, 4, and 6* a discussion of the replacement of vital nutrients is given.

Anemia: Chemotherapy can reduce the bone marrow's ability to make red blood cells, which carry oxygen to all parts of your body. When there are too few red blood cells, body tissues do not get enough oxygen to do their work. This condition is called anemia. Anemia can make you feel short of breath, very weak, and tired. It may be necessary to have the hormone EpoietinÒ and/or colony-stimulating factors to increase red cell or white cell levels. In addition, nutritional replacement therapy is essential to replace depleted stores of minerals, including iron.

Call your doctor if you have any of these symptoms:

- fatigue (feeling very weak and tired)

- dizziness or feeling faint

- shortness of breath

- feeling as if your heart is "pounding" or beating very fast

Your doctor will check you often during your treatment. She or he may also prescribe a medicine, such as *epigen* or *erythropoietin*, that can boost the growth of your red blood cells. Discuss this with your doctor if you become anemic often. If your red blood cell count falls too low, you may need a blood transfusion or a medicine called erythropoietin to raise the number of red blood cells in your body.

Things you can do if you are anemic:

- Get plenty of rest. Sleep more at night and take naps during the day if you can.

- Limit your activities. Do only the things that are essential or most important to you.

- Ask for help when you need it. Ask family and friends to pitch in with things like childcare, shopping, housework, or driving.

- Eat a well-balanced diet.

- When sitting, get up slowly. When lying down, sit first, and then stand. This will help prevent dizziness.

Reduction in white blood cells (WBCs) is also common in chemotherapy treatment. In these cases, great care must be taken to stay away from people with colds, the flu, or any other possible threatening infection. In cases where WBCs are low, a biological drug called *Neupogen* (colony stimulating factor) is given to increase the number of white blood cells.

Central nervous system problems: Chemotherapy can interfere with certain functions in your central nervous system (brain), causing tiredness, confusion, and depression. These feelings will go away, once the chemotherapy dose is lowered or you finish chemotherapy. Call your doctor if these symptoms occur.

Infection: Chemotherapy can make you more likely to get infections. This happens because most anticancer drugs affect the bone marrow, making it harder to make WBCs, the cells that fight many types of infections. Your doctor will check your blood cell count often while you are getting chemotherapy. As previously mentioned, Neupogen® (colony stimulating factor) is used to raise the WBC level to reduce the risk of infection. Most infections come from bacteria normally found on your skin and in your mouth, intestines, and genital tract. Sometimes, the cause of an infection may not be known. Even if you take extra care, you still may get an infection. But there are some things you can do. Antibiotics may be prescribed to help fight off the infection. Intravenous nutritional therapy can help decrease the risk of infection because it works to strengthen the immune system. In addition, probiotic support may be extremely beneficial in antibacterial support.

How can I help prevent infections?

- Wash your hands often during the day. Be sure to wash them before you eat, after you use the bathroom, and after touching animals.

- Clean your rectal area gently but thoroughly after each bowel movement. Ask your doctor or nurse for advice if the area becomes irritated or if you have hemorrhoids. Also, check with your doctor before using enemas or suppositories.

- Stay away from people who have illnesses you can catch, such as a cold, the flu, measles, or chicken pox.

- Try to avoid crowds. For example, go shopping or to the movies when the stores or theaters are least likely to be busy.

- Stay away from children who recently have received "live virus" vaccines, such as chicken pox and oral polio, since they may be contagious to people with a low blood cell count. Call your doctor or local health department if you have any questions.

- Do not cut or tear the cuticles of your nails.

- Be careful not to cut or nick yourself when using scissors, needles, or knives.

- Use an electric shaver instead of a razor to prevent breaks or cuts in your skin.

- Maintain good mouth care.

- Do not squeeze or scratch pimples.

- Take a warm (not hot) bath, shower, or sponge bath every day. Pat your skin dry using a light touch. Do not rub too hard.

- Use lotion or oil to soften and heal your skin if it becomes dry and cracked.

- Clean cuts and scrapes right away and daily with warm water, soap, and an antiseptic until healed.

- Avoid contact with animal litter boxes and waste, birdcages, and fish tanks.

- Avoid standing water, such as birdbaths, flower vases, or humidifiers.

- Wear protective gloves when gardening or cleaning up after others, especially small children.

- Do not get any immunizations, such as flu or pneumonia shots, without checking with your doctor first.

- Do not eat raw fish, seafood, meat, or eggs.

These recommendations can improve your quality of life while on chemotherapy and facilitate the healing process. The above recommendations are consistent with the National Cancer Institute.

Radiation Therapy

There are many forms of radiotherapy, with varied results. Not all regimens are the same. It is always prudent to implement integrative treatment to combat the negative effects of radiation. You may not be settled with radiotherapy, or you may be unsure as to whether it is right for you. This is why it is vital to research and get the expert advice from your oncologist and alternative health care physician before making a decision.

Radiotherapy, also called radiation therapy, is the treatment of cancer and other diseases with ionizing radiation. Ionizing radiation deposits energy that injures or destroys cells in the area being treated (the "target tissue") by damaging their genetic material, making it impossible for these cells to continue to grow. Although radiation damages both cancer cells and normal cells, the latter are able to repair themselves and function properly.

Radiotherapy may be used to treat localized solid tumors, such as cancers of the skin, tongue, larynx, brain, breast, or uterine cervix. It can also be used to treat leukemia (cancer of the blood-forming cells) and lymphoma (cancer of the lymphatic system). One type of radiation therapy commonly used involves photons or "packets" of energy. X-rays were the first form of photon radiation to be used to treat cancer. Depending on the amount of energy they possess, the rays can be used to destroy cancer cells on the surface of, or deeper in, the body. The higher the energy of the X-ray beam, the deeper the X-rays can go into the target tissue. Linear accelerators and betatrons are machines that produce X-rays of increasingly greater energy. The use of machines to focus radiation (such as X-rays) on a cancer site is called external beam radiotherapy.

Gamma rays are another form of photons used in radiotherapy. Gamma rays are produced spontaneously as certain elements (such as radium, uranium, and cobalt 60) and release radiation as they decompose or decay. Each element decays at a specific rate and gives off energy in the form of gamma rays and other particles. X-rays and gamma rays have the same effect on cancer cells.

Another technique for delivering radiation to cancer cells is to place radioactive implants directly in a tumor or body cavity. This is called internal radiotherapy. (Brachytherapy, interstitial irradiation, and intracavitary irradiation are types of internal radiotherapy.) In this treatment, the radiation dose is concentrated in a small area, and the patient stays in the hospital for a few days. Internal radiotherapy is frequently used for cancers of the tongue, uterus, and cervix. Several new approaches to radiation therapy are being evaluated to determine their effectiveness in treating cancer. One such technique is intra-operative irradiation, in which a large dose of external radiation is directed at the tumor and surrounding tissue during surgery.

Another investigational approach is particle beam radiation therapy. This type of therapy differs from photon radiotherapy in that it involves the use of fast-moving subatomic particles to treat localized cancers. A very sophisticated machine is needed to produce and accelerate the particles required for this procedure. Some particles (neutrons, pions, and heavy ions) deposit more energy along the path they take through tissue than do X-rays or gamma rays, thus causing more damage to the cells they hit. This type of radiation is often referred to as high linear energy transfer (high LET) radiation.

Scientists also are looking for ways to increase the effectiveness of radiation therapy. Two types of investigational drugs are being studied for their effect on cells undergoing radiation. Radiosensitizers make the tumor cells more likely to be damaged, and radioprotectors protect normal tissues from the effects of radiation. Hyperthermia, the use of heat, is also being studied for its effectiveness in sensitizing tissue to radiation. Other recent radiotherapy research has focused on the use of radiolabeled antibodies to deliver doses of radiation directly to the cancer site (radioimmunotherapy). Antibodies are highly specific proteins that are made by the body in response to the presence of antigens (substances recognized as foreign by the immune system).

Some tumor cells contain specific antigens that trigger the production of tumor-specific antibodies. Large quantities of these antibodies can be made in the laboratory and attached to radioactive substances (a process known as radiolabeling). Once injected into the body, the antibodies actively seek out the cancer cells, which are destroyed by the cell-killing (cytotoxic, or toxic to the cell) action of the radiation. This approach can minimize the risk of radiation damage to healthy cells. The success of this technique will depend upon both the identification of appropriate radioactive substances and determination of the safe and effective dose of radiation that can be delivered in this way.

Radiation therapy may be used alone or in combination with chemotherapy or surgery. Like all forms of cancer treatment, radiation therapy can have side effects. Possible side effects of treatment with radiation include temporary or permanent loss of hair in the area being treated, skin irritation, temporary change in skin color in the treated area, and tiredness. Other side effects are largely dependent on the area of the body that is treated.

What Are the Side Effects of Treatment?

External radiation therapy does not cause your body to become radioactive. There is no need to avoid being with other people because you are undergoing treatment. Most side effects of radiation therapy are related to the area that is being treated. Many patients have no side effects at all. Your doctor and nurse will tell you about the possible side effects you might expect and how you should deal with them. You should contact your doctor or nurse if you have any unusual symptoms during your treatment, such as coughing, sweating, fever, or pain.

The side effects of radiation therapy, although unpleasant, are usually not serious and can be controlled with medication or diet. They usually go away within a few weeks after treatment ends, although some side effects can last longer. Always check with your doctor or nurse about how you should deal with side effects. Throughout your treatment, your doctor will regularly check on the effects of the treatment. You may not be aware of changes in the cancer, but you probably will notice decreases in pain, bleeding, or other discomfort. You may continue to notice further improvement after your treatment is completed.

Your doctor may recommend periodic tests and physical exams to be sure that the radiation is causing as little damage to normal cells as possible. Depending on the area being treated, you may have routine blood tests to check the levels of red blood cells, white blood cells, and platelets, because radiation treatment can cause decreases in the levels of different blood cells.

What can I do to take care of myself during therapy?
Each patient's body responds to radiation therapy in its own way. That's why your doctor must plan and sometimes adjust your treatment. In addition, your doctor or nurse will give you suggestions for caring for yourself at home that are specific for your treatment and the possible side effects. Nearly all cancer patients receiving radiation therapy need to take special care of themselves to protect their health and to help the treatment succeed. Some guidelines to remember are given below.

- Before starting treatment, be sure your doctor knows about any medicines you are taking and if you have any allergies. Do not start taking any medicine (whether prescription or over-the-counter) during your radiation therapy without first telling your doctor or nurse.

- Fatigue is common during radiation therapy. Your body will use a lot of extra energy over the course of your treatment, and you may feel very tired.

- Be sure to get plenty of rest and sleep as often as you feel the need. It's common for fatigue to last for four to six weeks after your treatment has been completed.

- Good nutrition is very important. Try to eat a balanced diet that will prevent weight loss.

- Check with your doctor who specializes in natural medicine before taking nutritional and herbal preparations during treatment.

- Avoid wearing tight clothes, such as girdles or close-fitting collars, over the treatment area.

- Wear loose, soft cotton clothing over the treated area.

- Do not wear starched or stiff clothing over the treated area.

- Be extra kind to your skin in the treatment area.

- Ask your doctor or nurse if you may use soaps, lotions, deodorants, sun blocks, medicines, perfumes, cosmetics, talcum powder, or other substances in the treated area.

- Do not scratch, rub, or scrub treated skin.

- Do not use adhesive tape on treated skin. If bandaging is necessary, use paper tape and apply it outside the treatment area. Your nurse can help you place dressings, so that you can avoid irritating the treated area.

- Do not apply heat or cold (heating pad, ice pack, etc.) to the treated area. Use only lukewarm water for bathing the area.

- Use an electric shaver if you must shave the treated area but only after checking with your doctor or nurse. Do not use pre-shave lotions or hair removal products on the treated area.

- Protect the treatment area from the sun. Do not apply sunscreens just before a radiation treatment. If possible, cover treated skin with light clothing before going outside. Ask your doctor if you should use a sunscreen or a sun-blocking product. If so, select one with a protection factor of at least fifteen and re-apply it often. Ask your doctor or nurse how long after your treatments are completed you should continue to protect the treated skin from sunlight.

If you have questions, ask your doctor or nurse. They are the only ones who can properly advise you about your treatment, its side effects, home care, and any other medical concerns you may have. These recommendations can improve your quality of life while electing to do chemotherapy/radiotherapy and facilitate the healing process. The above recommendations are consistent with the National Cancer Institute.

Proton Therapy for Prostate Cancer (Adapted from Loma Linda Web site www.llu.edu)

Loma Linda University's Proton Treatment Center is the first proton facility in the world designed for patient treatment and research in a hospital setting. Protons improve physicians' ability to control beam delivery and to treat cancer and some benign disorders more effectively with radiation. More precise beam delivery increases the probability of disease control and reduces radiation received by normal tissues. Unnecessary radiation in normal tissues causes unwanted side effects and limits the use of conventional radiation (X-rays and electron beams).

Loma Linda physicians and scientists are specialists in proton radiation therapy, which has been shown to improve control of a variety of cancers and benign disorders. We have proven that protons can be used effectively and economically in a hospital setting where patients can be treated by a team of experts. At Loma Linda, we use protons for patients who have localized cancers of the brain, eye, head and neck, spinal cord, lung, abdomen, pelvis, prostate, and other sites. We also use protons for non-cancerous disorders, such as some forms of macular degeneration of the eye, arteriovenous malformations in the brain, and benign brain tumors.

We continually evaluate other conditions and anatomic sites and are studying ways to combine protons with other forms of treatment. We investigate, develop, and deliver high-quality proton treatments. We work closely with Loma Linda University Medical Center and Loma Linda University Cancer Institute to support the physical, emotional, and spiritual circumstances of patients and their families. We collaborate with others, such as the National Aeronautics and Space Administration (NASA), to seek better ways to use protons for treatment. In all of our work, we at the Proton Treatment Center support the mission of Loma Linda University and Medical Center: To Make Man Whole.

●●●

Chapter 8

Biological Therapy and Alternative Immunotherapy

The body has a natural ability to protect itself against diseases, including cancer. Biological and immunotherapy demonstrate remarkable results in cancer treatment.

B iological therapy (sometimes called immunotherapy, biotherapy, or biological response modifier therapy) is a promising new addition to the family of cancer treatments that includes surgery, chemotherapy, and radiation therapy. There is a vast amount of research and human studies that demonstrate the efficacy of these agents. It is always prudent to compare the studies and not hastily pursue immunotherapy and biological therapy. Asking your oncologist about these therapies is probably the best starting place.

What is Biological Therapy?

Biological therapies use the body's immune system, either directly or indirectly, to fight cancer or to lessen side effects that may be caused by some cancer treatments. The immune system, a complex network of cells and organs that work together to defend the body against attacks by "foreign," or "non-self" invaders, is one of the body's main defenses against disease. Researchers have found that the immune system may recognize the difference between healthy cells and cancer cells in the body and eliminate those that become cancerous. Cancer may develop when the immune system breaks down or is overwhelmed.

Biological therapies are designed to repair, stimulate, or enhance the immune system's natural anticancer function. Immune system cells and proteins, called antibodies, are part of the immune system and work against cancer and other diseases by creating an immune response against foreign invaders (antigens). This immune response is unique because antibodies are specifically programmed to recognize and defend against certain antigens. Antibodies respond to antigens by latching on to, or binding with, antigens, fitting together much the way a key fits a lock. Immune system cells work against disease, including cancer, in a variety of ways. Immune cells include the following:

- Lymphocytes, the main type of immune cell, are white blood cells found in the blood as well as in many other parts of the body. Lymphocytes include B cells, T cells, and NK cells.

- B cells (B lymphocytes) mature into plasma cells that secrete antibodies (immunoglobulins), proteins that recognize and attach to antigens.

- T cells (T lymphocytes) directly attack targeted foreign invaders. T cells direct and regulate the immune response by signaling other immune system defenders. T cells produce proteins called lymphokines, which are one type of cytokine. Cytokines are powerful chemical substances that control a number of cell activities, including the immune response.

- NK cells (natural killer cells) destroy cancer cells by producing powerful chemical substances that bind to and kill any foreign invaders.

- Monocytes are white blood cells that travel into tissues and develop, when needed, into macrophages, or "big eaters," as part of the immune response. Monocytes and macrophages play a key role in phagocytosis, a process by which some cells "eat" other cells and foreign invaders. Biological therapies, used to treat cancer, target some of these defenses, boosting, directing, or restoring the body's own cancer-fighting mechanisms.

Biological Response Modifiers

Substances used in biological therapies are often called biological response modifiers (BRMs). BRMs alter the interaction between the body's immune defenses and cancer, thus improving the body's ability to fight the disease. BRMs (such as cytokines and antibodies) are substances that occur naturally in the body. Scientists can now make BRMs in the laboratory that imitate or influence natural immune response agents. BRMs can play many roles in cancer treatment, including directly inhibiting tumor cell growth and acting indirectly to help healthy cells, particularly immune cells, control cancer. BRMs may be used to:

- enhance a cancer patient's immune system to fight cancer cell growth;

- eliminate, regulate, or suppress body responses that permit cancer growth;

- make cancer cells more susceptible to destruction by the immune response;

- alter cancer cells' growth patterns to promote behavior like that of healthy cells;

- block or reverse the process that changes a normal cell or a precancerous cell into a cancerous cell;

- enhance a cancer patient's ability to repair normal cells damaged by other forms of cancer treatment, such as chemotherapy or radiation; and

- prevent a cancer cell from spreading to other sites in the body.

Researchers are currently investigating a variety of BRMs, and many are being used in cancer treatment. These agents include interferons, interleukins, tumor necrosis factor, colony-stimulating factors, monoclonal antibodies, and cancer vaccines. These BRMs may prove to be most beneficial when used in combination with each other and/or with other treatments such as radiation and chemotherapy.

> **The interferons (IFN):** Interferons are types of cytokines that occur naturally in the body. They were the first cytokines produced in the laboratory for use as BRMs. While there are three major families of interferons, including interferon alpha, interferon beta, and interferon gamma, interferon alpha currently is the most widely used in cancer treatment. Researchers have found that interferons can improve a cancer patient's immune response against cancer cells. In addition, interferons may act directly on cancer cells by inhibiting their growth or promoting their development into cells with more normal behavior. Researchers believe that some interferons also may stimulate B cells and T cells, strengthening the immune system's anticancer function.
>
> The Food and Drug Administration (FDA) has approved the use of a type of interferon alpha for the treatment of certain types of cancer, including hairy cell leukemia, Kaposi's sarcoma (a rare cancer of cells lining blood vessels that often occurs in patients with AIDS), and chronic myelogenous leukemia, making it the first, but not the only, BRM approved for cancer therapy. Studies have shown that interferon alpha may also be effective in treating other cancers such as renal cell carcinoma (a type of kidney cancer) and some non-Hodgkin's lymphomas (cancers

that develop in the lymph system). When using interferons, combined with other BRMs or with chemotherapy, researchers are looking for improved treatments for these and other cancers in clinical trials (treatment studies). Investigators are exploring combinations of interferon alpha and chemotherapy to treat a number of cancers, including colorectal cancer (cancer of the bowel), multiple myeloma (cancer that effects bone marrow and bone), and melanoma (cancer that effects the skin).

Interleukins (IL): Like interferons, interleukins are cytokines that occur naturally in the body and can be made in the laboratory. Although many interleukins (including IL-1 through IL-15) have been identified, interleukin-2 (IL-2) has been the most widely studied in cancer treatment. IL-2 stimulates the growth and activities of many immune cells, such as lymphocytes, that can destroy cancer cells. Lymphocytes stimulated by IL-2, called lymphokine-activated killer (LAK) cells, have proven to be effective in destroying tumors.

Lymphocytes can be removed from a cancer patient's blood, stimulated with IL-2 in the laboratory, and returned to the patient as LAK cells, with the goal of improving the patient's anticancer immune response. Patients with advanced renal cell carcinoma or advanced melanoma have shown the best response to IL-2 therapy. In 1992, the FDA approved IL-2 for treating advanced metastatic renal cell carcinoma (kidney cancer that has spread).

Researchers are investigating the benefits of IL-2, used alone or with other treatments, in other cancers, such as colorectal cancer, ovarian cancer, and small-cell lung cancer in ongoing clinical trials. Combinations of IL-2 with other treatment methods, such as chemotherapy, surgery, or other BRMs, are also under study. Some scientists believe that IL-2 therapy may help stop certain cancers from growing, which can improve the length and quality of life for some cancer patients. Other interleukins, including IL-3, IL-4, IL-6, and IL-12, are also being studied. IL-12 has been demonstrating some impressive effects in melanoma. It is has shown to facilitate apoptosis (programmed cancer cell death) in melanoma laden cells.

Tumor Necrosis Factor (TNF): Tumor necrosis factor (TNF) is another type of cytokine under study. Like the interferons and interleukins, TNF stimulates the body's immune cells to fight cancer. TNF also directly affects tumor cells, damaging them and the blood vessels within the cancer. Without an adequate blood supply, a cancer cannot thrive. However, researchers are still uncertain exactly how TNF destroys tumors. Although TNF has shown promising anti-tumor activity in laboratory studies, the dose needed for this level of activity is extremely toxic. Researchers have found that TNF therapy is most effective and least toxic when directed at a specific tumor site, rather than administered throughout the body. Clinical trials are under way to investigate the effectiveness of TNF therapy alone and in combination with other BRMs in treating a variety of cancers.

Colony-Stimulating Factors (CSFs): Unlike TNF, colony-stimulating factors (CSFs) (sometimes called hematopoietic growth factors) usually do not directly affect tumor cells. Researchers have identified several CSFs (such as G-CSF and GM-CSF) that encourage bone marrow cells to divide and develop into various specialized white blood cells, platelets, and red blood cells. Bone marrow is important to the body's immune system because it is the source of all blood cells. The CSFs' stimulation of the immune system may benefit patients undergoing cancer treatment. Studies have shown that CSFs have the potential to:

- protect or restore bone marrow function when combined with chemotherapy or radiation, thus permitting the patient to tolerate higher doses of conventional anticancer therapy;

- aid in separating cancer cells from bone marrow that scientists have removed from the patient's body;

- stimulate immune system components, enhancing anti-tumor activity of other therapies; and

- help treat infections and other problems that may occur in patients who have received chemotherapy or in those whose immune systems are impaired.

Researchers have found CSFs particularly beneficial when used in combination with high-dose chemotherapy. Because anticancer drugs can damage the body's ability to make white blood cells, which are responsible for fighting infection, patients have an increased risk of developing infections during chemotherapy. Doctors must carefully monitor white blood cell levels during chemotherapy. However, using CSFs, which stimulate white blood cell activity, doctors can give higher, perhaps more effective, chemotherapy doses with decreased risk of infection. Because their immune system has been damaged, people who have had a bone marrow transplant are particularly susceptible to infections after the transplant. Doctors are evaluating the use of CSFs given to bone marrow transplant patients. Researchers have found that CSFs help blood cells in the immune system repair themselves more quickly after transplant, shortening the patient's recovery time and hospital stay.

Monoclonal Antibodies (MOABs): Researchers are evaluating the effectiveness of certain antibodies made in the laboratory, called monoclonal antibodies (MOABs). MOABs are specific for a particular antigen, and researchers are investigating ways to create MOABs specific to antigens found on cancer cells. Researchers make MOABs by injecting human cancer cells into mice so that their immune systems will make antibodies against these cancer cells. Researchers remove the mouse cells that are producing these antibodies and fuse them with a laboratory-grown immortal cell to create a "hybrid" cell called a hybridoma. Hybridomas are like factories that can indefinitely produce large quantities of these pure antibodies, or MOABs. MOABs may be used in cancer treatment in a number of ways:

- MOABs that react with specific types of cancer may enhance a patient's immune response to the cancer.

- MOABs may be linked to anticancer drugs, radioactive substances (radioisotopes), BRMs, or other toxins. When the antibodies latch onto cancer cells, they deliver these poisons directly to the tumor, helping to destroy it.

- Radioisotope-labeled MOABs may also prove useful in diagnosing certain cancers.

- MOABs may help destroy any cancer cells in a patient's bone marrow before an autologous bone marrow transplant in which bone marrow is removed from a patient, stored, and later given back to the patient after high-dose chemotherapy and/or radiation therapy.

MOABs are currently being tested in clinical trials in patients with lymphomas, colorectal cancer, lung cancer, leukemia, and a rare childhood cancer called neuroblastoma. Because the MOABs originally produced from hybridomas were foreign (mouse) proteins, patients often developed an immune response to them, producing human anti-mouse antibodies (HAMA). Newer MOABs have been engineered to minimize this problem.

Tumor vaccines: Tumor vaccines are another form of biological therapy currently under study. Vaccines for various diseases are effective because the immune system can develop acquired immunity to disease after initial exposure to it. This occurs because when T cells and B cells are activated, some of them become memory cells. The next time the same antigen enters the body, the immune system remembers how to destroy it. Researchers are developing tumor vaccines that may encourage the immune system to recognize cancer cells in this way. Tumor vaccines may help the body reject tumors and also help prevent cancer from recurring. Researchers are also investigating ways that tumor vaccines can be used in combination with BRMs. Tumor vaccines are being studied in treating melanoma, renal cell cancer, colorectal cancer, breast cancer, prostate cancer, and lymphomas.

Side Effects

Like other forms of cancer treatment, biological therapies can cause various side effects, which can vary widely from patient to patient. Because BRMs are often administered by injection, rashes or swelling may develop at the site where the shots are given. Several BRMs, including interferons and interleukins, may cause flu-like symptoms, including fever, chills, tiredness, and digestive tract problems. Blood pressure may also be affected. Side effects with IL-2 and TNF can often be severe, and patients need to be closely monitored during treatment. Side effects with antibody therapy vary, and allergic reactions may occur. Cancer vaccines may cause minor side effects, including fever and muscle aches. Some other specific effects may include:

- Flu-like symptoms including fever, chills, malaise, myalgia, and joint aches.

- Vascular leak syndrome.

- Usual dose-limiting toxicity, characterized by weight gain, arrhythmias, and/or tachycardia, low blood pressure, swelling and water retention, oliguria and renal insufficiency, pleural effusions, and pulmonary congestion.

- Suppresses bone marrow, anemia, thrombocytopenia, and neutropenia.

- Liver toxicity, elevated liver enzymes. Usually reversible within six to ten days after discontinuation of the drug.

- Skin rash.

- Thyroid alteration and other endocrine disturbance.

- Insomnia, depression, and impaired memory function.

- Infusion-related symptoms, including fever, chills, nausea and vomiting, urticaria, skin rash, fatigue, headache, diarrhea, dyspnea, and/or hypotension. Usually occur within the first week of initiation of therapy.

- Significant immunosuppressive agent with an increased incidence of opportunistic infections, including *Pneumocystis carinii*, cytomegalovirus (CMV), herpes zoster, *Candida, Cryptococcus,* and *Listeria* meningitis. Prophylaxis with anti-infective agents is indicated as outlined above. Recovery of CD4+ and CD8+ counts is slow and may take over one year to return to normal.

- Myelosuppression with neutropenia is most common, but anemia and thrombocytopenia are also observed. In rare instances, pancytopenia with marrow hyoplasia occurs, which can be fatal.

Special Precautions

- Use with caution on patients with preexisting cardiac, pulmonary, central nervous system (CNS), hepatic, and/or renal impairment, as there is an increased risk for developing serious and sometimes fatal reactions.

- Pretreatment evaluation should include complete blood counts (CBCs); serum chemistries, including liver function tests (LFTs), renal function, and electrolytes; pulmonary function tests (PFTs); and stress thallium.

- Patients should be monitored closely throughout the entire treatment, including vital signs every two to four hours, strict input and output, and daily weights. Continuous cardiopulmonary monitoring is important during therapy.

- Monitor for capillary leak syndrome (CLS), which begins almost immediately after initiation of therapy. Manifested by low blood pressure, peripheral edema, ascites, pleural and/or pericardial effusions, weight gain, and altered mental status.

- Toxic in pregnancy.

CLINICAL TRIALS

Details about clinical trials involving these and other biological therapies are available from PDQ, a National Cancer Institute (NCI) database of cancer information. Patients can ask their doctor to use PDQ, or they can call the NCI-supported Cancer Information Service (CIS) to request information about biological therapies and clinical trials.

ALTERNATIVE IMMUNOTHERAPY

It is important to recognize that immune enhancement therapy heightens immune surveillance. It is essential that the immune system recognizes itself as a friend and not as an enemy. This will allow for a defense response to the invader rather than healthy cells and systems. There is a communication that occurs between cells and the immune system. This communication is vital and, when enhanced, can improve the environment within the blood and body tissues. The Issels' and autologous vaccine are examples of powerful types of immunotherapy. There are many immune-modulating therapies that have beneficial effects in cancer treatment. In this book we will discuss the most prominent.

ISSELS' VACCINE

Josef M. Issels, MD, a German physician who laboriously worked with a countless number of patients and was influential in laying the groundwork for establishing several clinics in Europe, has become internationally known for his remarkable rate of complete, long-term remissions of "incurable cancers" (such as advanced cancers of the breast, uterus, prostate, colon, liver, lung, brain, sarcomas, lymphomas, and leukemias) in patients who had exhausted all standard treatments. After completion of the Issels' Treatment, these patients remained cancer-free for up to forty-five years, leading normal, healthy lives. The Issels' Treatment also significantly reduced the incidence of recurrent cancer after surgery, radiation, and chemotherapy, thereby considerably improving cure rates. The Issels' Treatment was able to reverse chronic degenerative diseases such as arthritis, lupus, Grave's disease, Sjoegren's syndrome, asthma, etc.

In 1951, Dr. Issels founded the first hospital in Europe for comprehensive immunotherapy of cancer. He was the medical director and director of research. In 1970, the hospital was enlarged from 80 to 120 patient beds. It contained extensive research facilities, including immunological and microbiological laboratories. The hospital's programs included research on tumor vaccines, mycoplasma vaccines, and bacterial vaccines, inducing fever, hyperthermia, etc. Ninety percent of the patients treated at the hospital had exhausted standard cancer treatment. From 1981 until 1987, Dr. Issels served as an expert member of, and advisor to, the Commission of the German Federal Government in the Fight Against Cancer. Dr. Issels presented many papers to national and international medical congresses and within programs of continuing education. He also published three monographs.

To summarize a complex form of treatment, the Issels vaccine is developed from the patient's own serum and processed with its own natural immune factors. The vaccine is made by culturing the patient's blood for several days and then isolating the stealth pathogens and their constituents and filtrating the endotoxins and purifying the serum. The serum is then re-injected into the patient subcutaneously. This injection causes an immune reaction by stimulating cytokine activity against the tumor. In addition, host immune defenses are heightened to fight against the cancer. Details about the Issels vaccine can be read about in Dr. Issels book, *Cancer: A Second Opinion*, or on line at issels.com.

Autologous Vaccine

There are other vaccines that are made from the patient's blood and variation, which include processing the vaccine with agents like 5-Aminopolypeptide and IL-12. The process of development is similar to the Issels vaccine. Again, the vaccine is known to stimulate cytokine and host immune defense. Dendrion is making a vaccine that is used in breast, multiple myeloma, and prostate cancer. However, this vaccine processes differently and utilizes donor tissue. More advances need to be made in vaccine therapy and the future is hopeful.

Antineoplastons

The most exciting and promising new direction of cancer research is in the body's own natural defense systems against cancer. Dr. Burzynski's work on the development of antineoplastons is both fascinating and miraculous. He has, through the last two decades, made incredible progress in developing this promising therapy. He received FDA approval to enter clinical trials and administer the treatment to selected candidates.

Most cancer experts believe we all develop cancer hundreds, if not millions, of times in our lifetimes. Given the trillions of developing cells, the millions of errors that can occur in the differentiating (maturing) process of each cell, and our constant exposure to carcinogenic substances (smoke, car fumes, radiation, etc.), the laws of probability dictate that mis-developing cells must occur frequently in the life of each individual. It stands to reason that a healthy body has a corrective system to "reprogram" newly-developed cancer cells into normal differentiation pathways before the cancer can take hold. Cancer cells differ from healthy cells in that they are, in effect, immortal. While healthy cells live a short while and then die, cancer cells continue dividing. The program for cell death is never activated.

Antineoplastons are peptides, small proteins and amino-acid derivatives, found naturally in human blood. Cancer patients tend to have low levels—as low as 2% that of healthy individuals. Antineoplastons work by "reprogramming" cancer cells to die like normal cells. Healthy cells are not affected. Antineoplastons have a two-pronged mechanism of activity. They suppress the activity of the oncogenes that cause cancer while at the same time stimulating the activity of the tumor-suppressor genes that stop cancer. There are specific peptides that are particularly effective against brain cancer and non-Hodgkin's lymphoma.

For further information, contact the Burzynski's Clinic web site at *www.cancermed.com*. This therapy is very expensive and current clinical trials lay heavy restrictions on who can and cannot receive the treatment. There is a waiting list and political process may not make it easy to access this potentially effective therapy.

Chapter 9

Hormone Replacement Therapy

The best word to describe whether or not hormone therapy is safe and effective in cancer treatment is caution.

There is much controversy over the use of hormone replacement therapy in the treatment of hormone-sensitive cancers (i.e., breast, uterine, and ovarian). Some believe that hormone replacement may be the right choice in opposing the action of the hormone that is causing cancer growth. In my opinion, it is essential that a thorough examination of hormone activity be accomplished as a part of the clinical work-up. In addition, hormone receptor assays give added information as to whether a cancer is expressing a particular hormone. This information is very important because it will help the clinician choose the appropriate therapy.

For example, an estrogen-receptor positive cancer is expressing a cancer fed by estrogen activity. This means that the cancerous tissue is positive for estrogen. Giving estrogen in treatment in this case would not be a prudent choice. There are cases where a cancer would express positive for both estrogen and progesterone. In this case, neither hormone should be used in therapy. The controversy is should hormones be used at all in cancer or do they, in

167

fact, demonstrate some benefit? An interesting article from WebMD medical news illustrates this point.

ESTROGEN USE MAY AFFECT BREAST CANCER TUMORS

Postmenopausal women who develop breast cancer are likely to have a less aggressive kind of tumor if they have previously taken estrogen, a new study suggests. Still, doctors say, the role medications may play in the development of breast cancer remains controversial. When women are diagnosed with breast cancer, they are given tests to establish the presence of estrogen receptors (ER) or progesterone receptors (PR) in the tumors. Tumors that are ER—or PR-positive tend to have a better prognosis and respond well to therapies such as tamoxifen. "We have known for some time that women diagnosed with breast cancer while taking extra hormones seem to have a better prognosis than those who are not," study author Elyse E. Lower, MD, tells WebMD. "In order to evaluate the impact of the biology of the tumor, we decided to look at estrogen and progesterone receptors as a marker. Having ER-positive tumors, which we found was associated with extra hormone usage, is a plus," Lower says. "That may help explain why those diagnosed with breast cancer while taking hormones actually have a better outcome." Lower, whose work was published in *Breast Cancer Research and Treatment,* is a professor of medicine at the University of Cincinnati College of Medicine. The researchers performed an analysis of all patients seen by one medical oncologist over a five-year period. Each patient's age, menopausal status, and the ER and PR content of her primary breast cancer were recorded. Patients were recorded as having taken "some" hormones if they had taken either birth control pills or hormone estrogen replacement therapy before their cancer diagnosis. Overall, breast cancers were ER-positive in 72% of the postmenopausal and 57% of the premenopausal women. Most of the patients had taken some form of hormone therapy. Postmenopausal patients who never took estrogen had a lower rate of ER-positive tumors (62%) than those who had (75%). The same relationship was seen for those with PR-positive tumors, which were found in 44% of those who had never used hormones and 58% of those who had. The difference was not statistically significant for premenopausal women, the researchers say. "We are not saying that women should be using estrogen because it will make your tumors less aggressive," Lower says. "Before, many women would be worried that because they were taking estrogen their tumors would be worse. Now we know the reason we don't see that is because estrogen probably does make the tumors biologically less aggressive." Further research is needed, says an expert who reviewed the study for WebMD. "Although they have established statistical significance, the clinical significance is not at all clear," Lind M. French, MD, tells WebMD. French is an associate professor in the department of family practice at the College of Human Medicine, Michigan State University, in Lansing. "It should also be pointed out that the majority of women in this study had ER in the tumors whether or not they had estrogen exposure. We really need a clinical trial before we can begin to make clinical recommendations."

—Kurt Ullman, RN WebMD Medical
News March 31, 2000
(Indianapolis)

Vital Information

- Breast cancer tumors that test positive for estrogen receptors (ER) and progesterone receptors (PR) are less aggressive and more responsive to treatment than those that do not.

- A new study shows that postmenopausal breast cancer patients who have a history of taking estrogen medications are more likely to have these ER—and PR-positive tumors.

- One expert says that the clinical significance of these findings remains unclear until further studies are done. At this time, the best word to describe whether or not hormone therapy is safe and effective in cancer treatment is *caution*. There is not enough research and conclusive evidence that the efficacy and safety are reliable. However, consider the alternatives. There are natural soy-based hormones that do not exhibit the same metabolic action as the synthetic brands, and there are many herbs that demonstrate phytohormonal properties that may be promising in cancer treatment.

- Herceptin receptor expression offers the new hope of receptor specific therapy.

> **Herceptin:** Herceptin is a monoclonal antibody that seeks out a specific target antigen known as HER2 receptors that lie on the surface of certain cancer cells. Women with breast cancer should be tested for the HER2 receptor site. Some women may express multiple copies of the gene that produces a protein HER2 growth factor, which plays a role in proliferation of cancer cells. In women that express HER2 protein, Herceptin binds to the cell and helps shrink the tumor. Herceptin has fewer side effects than traditional chemo agents. The most common adverse reaction is fever and chills and is usually not severe. Herceptin may cause damage to heart tissue and should be discontinued immediately if this has occurred.

> In the realm of appropriate testing for hormonal balance, there are saliva, urine, and blood tests available to give information on fractionated estrogens which include E1 (estrone), E2 (estradiol), and E3 (estriol, which is known as the protective form of estrogen), progesterone, testosterone, DHEA, and cortisol. It is advantageous to know the levels of these active hormones before initiating hormone replacement therapy. Should you have any further questions regarding hormone testing and therapy, consult your doctor who specializes in natural medicine.

Reduce Breast Cancer Risk

Oral contraceptives have shown to increase breast, uterine, and ovarian cancer risk. The longer oral contraceptives are used, the greater the risk. Other risk factors include family history of breast cancer, smoking, alcohol use, high fat and sugar in diet, inadequate nutrition, stress, and hormonal dysfunction.

How Do I Reduce the Risk Factors?

- Identify the risk factors. Some are mentioned above.

- Perform proper screening. Self-breast exam, mammogram, and ultrasound are effective ways of screening for cancer. These are first line tests that can detect early changes.

- Improve diet and lifestyle. Eat more fiber and greens, use juicing, eliminate or dramatically reduce the amount of red meat. Definitely be sure it is hormone-free meat. Reduce fat intake. Lose weight if this is a risk factor for you. Practice effective stress reduction and exercise.

Consider nutritional and herbal replacement. There are many protective nutrients and herbs that have anti-cancerous properties. Here is a partial list:

- CoQ10 (400 mg daily)

- Vitamins E and C (500 IU of E and 2000 mg of C three times a day)

- Milk thistle extract 600–1000 mg daily (prevents toxic accumulation of estrogens)

- Saw PALMETTO extract (anti-tumor immune enhancing effects)

- Boron (aids estrogen metabolism)

- Essential fatty acids (good fats that aid in strengthening the immune system)

- Calcium D-Glucarate (aids estrogen metabolism)

- Indole-3-Carbinol (400-800 mg daily) (anti-tumor and estrogen metabolism)

These are just a few items that demonstrate preventive properties. At the end of the book, there is a case study on breast cancer and a sample treatment plan without listing dosages. This is one among many cases that I have had opportunity to treat in my practice.

● ●

Chapter 10

Intravenous Chelation and Nutritional Therapy

Though cancer is often considered an incurable disease, blended treatment proves to be powerful and effective.

Intravenous therapy is becoming more popular in cancer treatment. This form of therapy focuses on nutritional replacement, anticancer action, chelation, and detoxification. The substances usually included in the IV solution are vitamins, minerals, amino acids, chelating compounds, and specialized biochemical medicines that are used to inhibit cancer activity. IV therapy usually takes one to two hours per session and is recommended twice weekly. This therapy is most often used as a complementary therapy, in addition to conventional cancer treatment.

CHELATION THERAPY

Chelation therapy in cancer is becoming more popular. The rationale behind using chelation therapy is mainly based in detoxification on a cellular level. Dr. Leon Chaitow explains this in his book on chelation therapy, *The Cancer Connection.*

By now, the concept of free radical damage, resulting in tissue damage and consequent deterioration of circulatory function, should be quite familiar. It is perhaps less apparent that free radical damage is frequently the trigger which leads to malignant changes in previously normal cells. Just as the first benefits to circulation of EDTA chelation therapy were discovered during treatment of heavy metal poisoning, so was the way in which this same treatment could help prevent, and indeed treat, cancer discovered. Writing in a Swiss medical journal in 1976, Dr. W. Blumen described the strange, but potentially very important, discovery. In the late 1950s, a group of residents of Zurich who lived adjacent to a major traffic route were treated for contamination by lead with EDTA chelation under the auspices of the Zurich Board of Health. These people had all inhaled large amounts of lead-laden fumes and were suffering from a range of symptoms identified as being related to lead poisoning, including stomach ache, fatigue, headache, digestive symptoms, etc. Lead deposits were found to be present in their gum tissues and specific changes were found in their urine, linking their condition with high lead levels. Some years later, in the early 1970s, people living in the same area were being investigated for the incidence of cancer in an attempt to link the pollution with a higher cancer rate than average. This link was easily established as fully 11 percent of the residents of the road had died of cancer over the period 1959 to 1972, a rate some 900 percent above that expected when compared with people living in the same community but not directly affected by lead pollution. The forms of cancer most commonly related involved the lungs, colon, stomach, breast, and ovary. But what of the people previously treated with EDTA back in 1959? Only 1 of the 47 people in that group had developed cancer. The cancer rate in people in the contaminated area who had not received EDTA was 600 percent above that of the group who had chelation. Far and away, the best protection from lead toxicity and its long-term effects is to avoid it altogether. However, this is, of course, not always within the control of the individual and a second best bet is to have the lead removed via chelation as a protective measure against its undoubted toxicity, which can contribute toward the evolution of cancer. Australian research scientist John Sterling, who has worked at the famous Issels clinic in Germany, mentions in a personal communication that Issels had noted a marked protective effect against cancer after use of EDTA chelation. Animal studies (using mice) have shown that intravenous EDTA plays a preventive role against cancer, largely, it is thought, through removal of metallic ions, which seem to be essential for tumor growth. Walker and Gordon believe that the prevention offered to the citizens of Zurich was partly as a result of removal of metal ions and of lead (which can chronically depress immune function) and also due to the improvement in circulation which chelation produced. Tumors flourish in areas of poor oxygenation and the increase in the levels of this, which chelation allows, would, they believe, be sufficient to retard cancer development. Halstead (1979) points to the significant increase in metal ions found as tissues age and the increased likelihood of cancer developing. There is also a proven link between high levels of certain metals in topsoil and cancer in the same regions. Interestingly, he confirms that most forms of chemotherapy involve drugs which have chelating effects either directly or as a result of breakdown of their constituents.

He quotes experimental studies which show that in some forms of cancer, such as Ehrlich's ascites tumor, the use of EDTA was significantly able to strip the tumor cells of their heavy protective coat, allowing other mechanisms (such as protein digesting enzymes) to destroy the tumors. At the very least, EDTA chelation can be seen to offer a useful line of investigation in cancer prevention, and possibly treatment, in some forms of this disease.

Chelation Therapy. Leon Chaitow, Leon N.D., D.O.

Chelation therapy is a promising adjunctive treatment in cancer. The dosage of EDTA administered depends on the height and weight and kidney clearance of the individual receiving treatment. Your doctor should calculate the EDTA dose based upon the above criteria before administering treatment. In addition, the chelation fluid should include the vitamins that enhance the therapy. Minerals should be replaced, following the administration of chelation fluid. Minerals are not included in the chelation fluid because of the chelating action against the minerals. If it is all given in one lump sum, the individual will not have adequate mineral replacement and can become deficient. Intravenous chelation can take from one and one-half to three hours to complete, and it is recommended that twenty to twenty-four consecutive treatments be administered.

Oral Chelation

There are some formulations that are said to work better than intravenous chelation therapy. It is debatable as to whether EDTA, DMSA, and DMPS are orally absorbed. These formulations may have a limited amount of efficacy. Clinical evaluation is necessary to determine efficacy. Based on my experience, I have observed laboratory markers, i.e. homocysteine, C-reactive protein, and lipids reduce. Furthermore, ultrasounds and coronary scans demonstrate reduced plaque and calcium deposits on arteries with intravenous chelation. I have not seen as an impressive result with oral formulations.

NUTRITIONAL REPLACEMENT THERAPY

Using IV therapy to replace nutritional deficiencies is an efficient method to ensure proper nutrition. This therapy is recommended in addition to conventional treatments. Nutritional replacement therapy offers many benefits to those on chemotherapy experiencing a loss of appetite during treatment. The substances usually included in the IV solution are vitamins, minerals, amino acids, and nutritional and/or herbal substances that enhance immune function. Nutritional IV replacement takes one hour to perform and is generally tolerated well by most patients. For further information on oral supplementation, the next chapter will discuss that and the essential nutrients in preventing and treating cancer. See Appendix #3 for an example of nutrients contained in IV support theropy.

Chapter 11

Nutritional and Diet Therapies

Most integrative treatment protocols begin with consideration of the patient's nutritional balance.

Nutritional deficiencies can make an individual vulnerable to cancer onset. Today, the food quality is compromised, and the concentration of nutrients in food is greatly reduced. When considering an integrative approach to cancer treatment, it is necessary to have nutritional supplementation as part of the overall plan. Below are some of the most important nutrients to consider.

Amino Acids

These are the building blocks of proteins and have specific action in cancer therapy. Free form amino acids should be administered orally or intravenously to enhance rebuilding of healthy cells and restoration and repair of tissue damaged during chemotherapy and radiation therapy.

ANTIOXIDANTS IN CANCER THERAPY

There is much confusion and conflicting information surrounding the use of antioxidants in conventional cancer treatments. This is reminiscent of the vitamin C controversy that occurred almost three decades ago and still continues to this day. With all the hoopla this controversy produces, Linus Pauling's monumental work has flourished, and there are thousands of research articles that establish the safe and effective use of vitamin C. A responsible evaluation of antioxidants and their safe use is what the general public needs, instead of an "us against them" scenario that only attracts negative publicity.

When a person is suffering with cancer, the illness in and of itself occupies every ounce of their physical and emotional stamina. The very last thing that is needed is a war between two systems of medicine that both have much to offer a person suffering with cancer, if appropriately blended. I have had patients come to me frustrated because there are two differing opinions regarding the use of antioxidants in cancer treatment. Oncologists have called my office and strongly disputed the use of antioxidants while a patient is undergoing chemotherapy and radiation therapy. In this case, I say, "the poor patient." The bottom line is this argument and confusion takes away from the healing energy and adds more stress to the individual and the environment. I firmly believe that antioxidant therapy is necessary in cancer treatment and should be administered in an integrated manner.

Let's nip it while we can. What are the concerns? There is concern that antioxidants reduce oxidizing free radicals, which are highly reactive molecules that are produced by chemotherapy and radiotherapy to destroy the cancer. This is thought to thereby decrease the effectiveness of chemotherapy and radiotherapy. This raises the question: Should antioxidants be used at all in cancer treatment? After reviewing some of the medical literature and observing the favorable results produced in my cancer patients, I have the following recommendations.

Should Antioxidants Be Used in Cancer Treatment?

After reviewing the evidence, I have found antioxidants to be beneficial in various cancers, if used appropriately. It is my opinion that too much of a good thing can have negative results. Balance and skill in using antioxidants are both necessary for the best outcome. Considerable data exists showing increased effectiveness of many cancer therapy agents, as well as a decrease in adverse effects, when antioxidants are given along with conventional treatment.

Antioxidants protect cell free radical-mediated damage. Research data have shown that free radicals frequently have a role in the process of cancer initiation and promotion. Free radicals are produced in normal cellular processes through the body's use of oxygen. Environmental factors such as smog, radiation, pesticides, herbicides, many drugs, and cigarette smoke can react within the body to cause free radical production. Unchecked by an antioxidant, the highly unstable free radicals attack cell constituents, including DNA and other opportune targets, particularly those containing polyunsaturated fatty acids. Free radicals can damage both the structure and function of cell membranes; nucleic acids and electron-dense regions of proteins also come under attack. Increased incidence of cancer with advancing age may be due, at least in part, to the increasing level of free radical reactions with age, along with the diminishing ability of the immune system to eliminate altered cells.

Antioxidant defense systems. Antioxidant defenses that help protect the body from free radical damage include the enzymes superoxide dismutase, catalase and glutathione peroxidase, vitamins C and E, carotenoids, alpha-lipoic acid, and bioflavonoids, such as are present in Pycnogenol® (pine bark extract).

179

Selenium, zinc, strontium, and vanadium also are involved in the complex antioxidant defense system and should be considered in the treatment of cancer.

Functions of nutrients used in cancer prevention. There is substantial evidence that many dietary factors influence the incidence of cancer in humans. Some nutrients alter cancer incidence and growth, acting as anti-carcinogens. Nutritional anti-carcinogens function in several ways.

They

1. inhibit tumor initiation by altering cell functions;

2. pick up active forms of carcinogens and prevent them from reaching target sites;

3. enhance the body's defense systems;

4. inhibit or reduce progression of previously initiated cancers;

5. prevent the activation of genes and the proliferation of cells by tumor promoters.

Information to date is relatively limited as to which nutrients in what concentrations are effective in preventing cancer in humans. Because of the different cells that become cancerous, as well as the number of agents that can cause human cancer, preventive measures may be effective for one cancer but not for another.

CURRENT CANCER RESEARCH

The following summary of current research on the antioxidants and cancer, using selected studies, is intended as a balanced overview. It demonstrates that the antioxidants show promise as cancer prevention agents, alone and in combination. Additional studies are under way in a number of countries to further investigate the role of the antioxidants in prevention and control of cancer. A number of actions of the antioxidants have relevance to their role in cancer prevention and control.

1. Vitamin A

   - Retinoic acid has demonstrated promising results in the treatment of leukemia.

   - Vitamin A and beta carotene increase radiation's effect in the body, and vitamin A improves response rates.

   - Vitamin A increases the response rates of specific chemo agents.

   - No evidence that vitamin A reduces the effects of chemotherapy or radiation.

2. Vitamin C

   - increases the effect of radiotherapy in humans;

   - increases the effects of specific chemo agents;

   - high concentrations can increase the resistance to doxirubicin in resistant breast cancer cells;

   - there is no evidence that vitamin C decreases the effects of chemotherapy or radiation.

3. Vitamin E

   - induces tumor cell death;

   - increases survival time when administered with omega-3 fatty acids in terminal cancer patients;

   - doses below 500 mg/kg may increase the effect of radiotherapy;

- increases the activity of specific chemo agents;

- there is no evidence exists that vitamin E reduces the effect of chemotherapy or radiation.

4. Selenium

- There is incomplete data in its effects in radiotherapy.

- Selenium increases activity in specific chemo agents and decreases toxicity.

- No evidence exists that suggests selenium reduces the effect of chemotherapy.

5. CoQ10

- inhibits tumor growth activity in breast cancer;

- works well as an adjunct to chemo agents;

- strengthens cell wall protection;

- there is no evidence of inhibitory effects in chemo-therapy and radiotherapy.

In addition to its role as a free radical scavenger, vitamin E at high levels enhances the body's immune response, which may play a role in cancer defenses. Vitamin E protects vitamin A from destruction in the body and spares selenium. Vitamin E also inhibits the conversion of nitrites—present in smoked, pickled, and cured foods—to nitrosamines in the stomach. Nitrosamines are cancer-causing agents. Vitamin C also prevents conversion of nitrites to nitrosamines and enhances the immune response. Vitamin A stimulates the immune response and controls the growth, alteration, and functions of body tissues.

Carotenoids are effective quenchers of singlet oxygen and function as chain-breaking antioxidants. Carotenoids enhance the immune response. Certain carotenoids (including lycopene and beta-carotene) can increase communication between cells. Increased communication between normal cells and cells that have been damaged by cancer-causing agents prevents the damaged cells from becoming malignant. Selenium, in addition to its inclusion in the enzyme glutathione peroxidase (which deactivates free radicals), enhances the immune response, resulting in potentially increased resistance to cancer initiation and growth.

Retinoic acid has demonstrated the ability to inhibit tumor growth and should be strongly considered as an adjunct to standard chemotherapeutics. Retinoic acid is said to increase the effectiveness of chemotherapy and prevent toxic reactions. Results to date: cell, animal, and epidemiologic studies suggest that the antioxidants may alter cancer incidence and growth by acting as anticarcinogens. Conversely, a dietary deficiency of the antioxidants may enhance the incidence of certain cancers.

It is important that an individual on a cancer treatment plan include healthy dietary goals, adequate fluid intake, nutritional and metabolic therapy, and immune therapy. Antioxidants should be part of this treatment strategy but not an isolated therapy. There are different treatment regimens for cancer, and when designing a program this must be considered. I would not advise mega-dosing antioxidants. With careful administration, antioxidants can heighten the effectiveness of the overall treatment plan.

Nutrients Demonstrating Protective Effects against Cancer

The following nutrients are listed in alphabetical order. For further detail on these nutrients and their efficacy in cancer, you can do an online search for each nutrient. You will discover that a significant amount of information is available. I just highlighted relevant information to whet your appetite.

Beta carotene: Carotenoids have protective effects against cancer. Vitamin A and beta carotene demonstrate immune-enhancing properties. This nutrient is the precursor to vitamin A. Vegetables (carrots, spinach, and leafy greens) are found to have high concentrations of both alpha and beta carotene. Both forms of carotene are important in nutrition and prevention of disease. Beta carotene has demonstrated useful protective effects in lung and cervical cancer. Supportive dose is 125 mg daily.

Beta-1 3 D-Glucan: This nutrient is considered to be a very potent immune modulator. Some prestigious medical schools, such as Harvard and Tulane universities, have extensively studied the immune-modulating effects of Beta-1 3 D-Glucan. This nutrient enhances immunity by stimulating macrophage activity and activating against free radical activity. It is also known to speed up tissue repair and destroy mutated cells that are the cause of many cancers. This substance is derived from baker's yeast and is safe to use, unless an individual has an allergy to baker's yeast.

Calcium: This mineral can protect against colon cancer. Calcium is essential in the formation of healthy bones and teeth. It is also extremely important in blood clotting and cellular metabolism. The foods that are rich in calcium include dark, leafy-green vegetables, nuts, seeds, and fish.

Chromium: Chromium has been found to be an extremely important trace nutrient in assisting thyroid metabolism and glucose regulation. Immune function improves and a higher resistance to cancer develops when blood sugar levels are regulated properly and balanced metabolic activity is achieved.

Colostrum: Colostrum is a nutritional substance that has demonstrated some promising immune modulating activity. It is the very first substance excreted in mother's milk and essential in laying the foundations of a strong immune system. The product quality varies according to origin of supply and manufacturing standards. In cancer therapy, it may be useful in providing immune enhancement and active immune defense against tumor growth. Colostrum is considered a biological nutritional, and there may be individuals who cannot take this product because of their sensitivity to it.

Copper: Copper is essential to healthy immune function. Copper is essential for healthy white blood cell and red blood cell activity and can fight against cancer. However, copper can also accumulate in body tissue in toxic amounts, causing immune suppression and fatigue. Maintaining body balance and addressing the body's needs are the keys to good health.

Folic Acid: This important nutrient is necessary in proper synthesis of RNA and DNA. It is a protective vitamin against some forms of cancer. Folic acid may become deficient during chemotherapy. Consult your physician on replacement guidelines. With certain chemotherapeutic agents (Methotrexate), folic acid may inhibit effectiveness and should not be administered in doses greater than 400-800 mcg daily, until chemotherapy sessions are completed.

Garlic: Garlic is a food that has been used for its medicinal properties for centuries. Garlic used in cancer treatment can lower the risk of tumor formation in the stomach, colon, lungs, and esophagus. If you don't have an allergy to garlic, then I suggest that you have it in your diet in copious amounts.

Germanium: This is a trace mineral that enhances the availability of oxygen to healthy cells and cancer cells. Cancer cells cannot survive well in an oxygen-rich environment. Germanium slows cancer growth and is recommended in any integrative cancer regimen.

Inositol: Inositol was found to be an important phytochemical that has demonstrated anti-cancer activity. It is classified as one of the B vitamins but really should be classified as a single nutrient. In the body, inositol helps remove excess fat from tissues. It is thought that within this fat accumulates toxins that aggravate cancer.

Iodine: This mineral has shown to be effective in protection against breast cancer. Iodine is necessary in promoting the growth and repair of body tissue.

IP-6: IP-6, also known as Phytopharmica's Cellular Forté, is the one and only patented combination of IP-6 and inositol that greatly increases natural killer-cell activity. Cellular Forté increases the level of inositol phosphates in the cells. This heightened activity dramatically increases natural killer-cell activity, which strengthens the entire immune system. When inositol combines with IP-6, they convert into two IP-3 molecules upon reaching the cells. These IP-3 molecules are essential for regulating healthy cell growth. The IP-6 molecule consists of Inositol and six phosphate groups. When this compound is combined with Inositol (no phosphate groups), IP-6 transfers three of its six phosphates to inositol, creating two IP-3s, once it reaches the body's cells. In cancer therapy, IP-6 is a potent immune modulator and should be included in the treatment regimen.

Magnesium: This is a general protective nutrient in cancer. Your heart and blood vessels need magnesium for healthy function. In addition, magnesium is needed to form healthy genetic material such as RNA and DNA.

Manganese: Manganese promotes healthy oxygen uptake, carbohydrate and fat metabolism, and is important in many enzyme systems. It also has direct action on white blood cells and their binding ability. Manganese is important in regulating a healthy immune system and should be included in the overall treatment plan for cancer.

MGN-3: MGN-3 is a powerful immune stimulator that enhances natural killer (NK) cell activity against tumor cells. The research demonstrates some promising results in cancer treatment. MGN-3 is used extensively in cases of multiple myeloma and in other cancers as well. In my opinion the efficacy of this agent remains to be seen. Further research and clinical trials are necessary to assure the public that MGN-3 does in fact demonstrate favorable clinical results.

Molybdenum: This trace mineral is required in small amounts. Deficiency of molybdenum is associated with increased cancer risk .

Omega 3, 6, and 9 Fatty Acids (EFAs): These are known as the good fats. They are very important in keeping body tissue healthy. According to some studies, these fatty acids may inhibit cancer activity, especially hormone-related cancers. A good, fresh supply of fish, flaxseed, sunflower, and borage oils are recommended for obtaining adequate EFAs. There are also freeze-dried powders available that may be more palatable and can be mixed in juice.

Potassium: Potassium can counteract cancer. By increasing the potassium concentration in the body, enhanced cellular function results, thereby decreasing the formation of cancerous tissue. Dr. Max Gerson found that raising potassium in the diet and increasing its concentrations in the body helped counteract tumor growth.

Probiotics (acidophilus, lactobacillus, etc.): These are known as the "friendly bacteria" that naturally inhabit the gastrointestinal tract. Probiotics are known to have protective properties against cancer in general. Probiotic activity is the direct opposite of antibiotic action. The antibiotics can wipe out all of the bowel flora. This can leave the bowel vulnerable to more pathogenic strains of bacteria. Probiotics specifically work on the bowel ecology, reducing disease-causing bacteria and toxic load, and raising the beneficial bacteria (acidophilus, bifidus, etc.). These beneficial bacteria are needed to provide the delicate balance. Probiotics are known to raise the immune activity in the bowel, thereby, contributing to the overall protection against cancer. Usually as a maintenance dose, I recommend one teaspoonful, one to two times daily. In active cancer, when infection is present, I prescribe a therapeutic dose.

Selenium: Selenium is a trace nutrient and is very important in antioxidant defense. Selenium supplementation has demonstrated tumor-inhibiting effects. When taking selenium, prescribed dosing must be followed, otherwise toxicity may result. Doses of 1,000 mcg of selenium have been known to cause loss of hair and adverse neurological symptoms.

Vitamin B6: This vitamin is found in leafy greens, bananas, and other fruit. It is essential for the healthy function of the immune system and overall protection against negative environmental factors such as pollution. It is needed for healthy function of the nervous system and is often consumed in high amount under stress. Supportive dose is no more than 200 mg daily.

Vitamin B12: Vitamin B12 is used in cases of pernicious anemia, which is an anemia of the blood. Vitamin B12 is necessary for healthy cell development. Chemotherapy and radiation often reduce the levels of B12 in the body tissues and blood. This vitamin should be given along with folic acid, and it is best to give intramuscular injections for better absorption. There are several forms of vitamin B12. The most commonly used form is known as cyanocobalamin. This form of vitamin B12 is not metabolically effective. Most patients who have tried this form of B12 say that they really haven't noticed any results. The preferred form of B12 is hydroxycobalamin, which is long lasting and metabolically active. Most of my patients notice an immediate energy increase and overall improvement in memory. The next form of B12 is known as methylcobalamin, which is even superior to hydroxycobalamin but also very expensive. I notice excellent results with this form of B12, but use it less frequently because of cost. Vitamin B12 should be included in your cancer treatment plan. The injections should also include folic acid. I recommend at least two injections per week.

Vitamin B Complex: Vitamin B complex includes thiamin, riboflavin, niacin, and pantothenic acid. All of these B vitamins are important in healthy immune function and glandular support. For healthy formation of body tissue, the B vitamins must be adequately supplied. Chemotherapy and radiation therapies deplete the body of these vitamins and it is essential that these vitamins be replaced.

Vitamin C: Vitamin C is the most widely studied and has many benefits associated with its use. Linus Pauling's work in the action of vitamin C is a benefit that will be with mankind for ages to come. Vitamin C is an important component in maintaining a healthy immune system and in protecting against many varieties of cancer. The dosing of vitamin C depends upon the individual's tolerance, therapeutic need, and utilization in the body. I recommend to all patients the use of vitamin C in their daily prevention regimen. Intravenous use of vitamin C is very effective in its cancer fighting and immune supportive properties. It is recommended to take no more than 10 grams daily. Supportive dosing is about 2000 mg three times daily.

Vitamin E: This vitamin is found in dark green vegetables, eggs, herbs, and some oils used in cooking. It is also found in organ meats. Vitamin E is known as a powerful antioxidant. It protects against oxidation caused by free radical activity in the body and strengthens body tissue. There are studies that demonstrate vitamin E's usefulness in protecting against bowel cancer. Supportive dose is 500–800 IU daily.

Water: Water is an essential nutrient necessary to all living organisms. Water is important in maintaining enzyme systems and detoxifying the body of waste products. A good, fresh purified source of water is a must for every human being. We should be very careful to guard and protect our water, for it is a precious element. It is very important while undergoing cancer treatment to keep your water intake upward of 1.5 liters daily.

Zinc: Zinc is known as a powerful immune-boosting mineral. Zinc is necessary to have healthy immune function. However, too much zinc can fatigue the immune system. Immune suppression may result if zinc is taken in excess of 60 mg daily. Zinc is an important mineral in protecting against cancer but must be used in proper dosing.

Diet Therapy and Nutrition

There are many different suggested diets for cancer therapy. Malnutrition is of major concern in cancer patients. Researchers estimate that the cause of death for 40% of cancer patients is from malnutrition. Improving dietary habits is an absolute necessity. However, it would be prudent, particularly in cancer treatment, to have as part of the health care team a nutritionist specializing in a whole-foods approach in healing. A general resource is a book entitled: *What to Eat If You Have Cancer: A Guide to Adding Nutritional Therapy to Your Treatment Plan,* written by Maureen Keane, Daniella Chace , John A. Lung. (NTC/Contemporary Publishing. ISBN 0-8092-3261-8.)

This book is a guide to adding nutritional therapy to traditional cancer treatment programs. It includes an overview of how cancer affects the body, current nutritional information, and meal planning suggestions that facilitate healing.

Another diet you may want more information on is the Gerson Diet. For detailed information concerning this diet, visit www.gerson.org on the Internet. Below is a segment taken from the *Gerson Healing Newsletter* written by Charlotte Gerson. After reading this excerpt, you will have a feel for the type of diet and therapy that is recommended for cancer treatment.

Gerson Patients' Problems

The following is excerpted in order for you to gain a better understanding of what commitment is required to follow all of the recommendations of the Gerson approach to healing. There are some individuals that do not have the innate ability to adhere to such a rigorous routine. However, there are countless number of cancers that have remitted as a result of this combination diet and whole body therapy.

It has frequently occurred to me that, in order to really be sure that the patients understand and follow the Gerson

191

Therapy exactly, I ought to follow them around their house and kitchen for twenty-four hours. A situation that arose recently amply illustrates the point. I was surprised and shocked by these deviations from the therapy; but, since they were taking place, I felt that it was necessary to share my concerns with our friends and other patients in order to make them aware and prevent errors. The patient in question was not only very much interested in the Gerson Therapy for his own recovery, he felt so strongly about spreading the word of healing that he organized a Gerson Convention Day. He also invited me to stay at his lovely home overnight, so that I could be spoiled with good, organic Gerson food and juices. The house is located in a wooded area, with beautiful huge trees, at the edge of a small lake. In other words, the air is clean and fresh and the atmosphere relaxing—no problem there. The patient's business is well organized and runs quite well with minimal attention, so he is able to get a lot of rest. There is help in the household, so there are no pressures in the juice and food preparation. But there are at least four major problems in the patient's application of the therapy.

1. The water is "hard"; it contains minerals. So, like other people in the area, the patient's home is equipped with "water softener" equipment. His very warm, concerned, and cooperative wife is doing everything in her power to help her husband recover. Yet she stated that she brings in "sacks of salt" for the water softener! As our readers know, in the process of removing the unwelcome minerals in the water, the equipment replaces these with sodium. What happens as a result is that the patient washes and bathes in "softened water," loaded with salt. Salt is very easily absorbed through the skin and should never be used by a Gerson patient. Salt is an enzyme inhibitor and the Gerson Therapy is designed to remove excess sodium. Salt is needed for fast growth of tumor tissue. It is also the basis of the "tissue damage syndrome," when normal cells lose

their ability to hold potassium while sodium penetrates, causing edema and loss of function. This tissue damage is, according to Dr. Gerson, the beginning of all chronic disease. Naturally, bathing in salt water must be avoided at all cost.

2. We were served a very delicious and attractive lunch, which included a lovely salad loaded with avocados. I immediately asked if the patient, too, was eating them. He was! This was another serious mistake, since avocados contain a fairly large percentage of fat. This is the reason why they are forbidden, because fats tend to stimulate new tumor growth! The lady of the house said that she thought that avocados were served at the Mexican Gerson Hospital—which they are not. The problem here is that the patient or caregiver should not rely on memory. All these items are clearly set down in *A Cancer Therapy*; and avocados are the second item on the "Forbidden" list. We have to ask patients and caregivers to read and re-read the "Therapy" chapter in the book, chapter XXXIII, p. 237, and make sure that they understand all the directions exactly and follow all instructions.

3. Along with the lunch, we had a very nice vegetable soup. It contained some zucchini, peas, celery, onions, and a few other vegetables. The patient asked me how I enjoyed the "Hippocrates Soup." I had to state that the soup we had was not Hippocrates soup, as Dr. Gerson describes it in the book. The combination of ingredients that are supposed to be in that soup are clearly described in *A Cancer Therapy* as well as the *Gerson Therapy Handbook* (formerly, *Gerson Therapy Primer*), and they are very specific. Hippocrates (the father of medicine) understood that this special combination of ingredients has a

beneficial, detoxifying effect on the kidneys. That is the reason why Dr. Gerson used it. He felt that this soup was so important that he wanted patients to eat the "special soup" twice daily to benefit the kidneys and help them clear toxins from the body. Occasionally, one can add extra tomatoes to give the soup a different flavor; or one can cut up and roast some onions on a dry cookie sheet (NO fat, butter, or oil) in the oven. Then these can be added to the same basic soup recipe for a tasty treat. However, the basic recipe should remain unchanged.

4. The lady of the house also thoughtfully offered me some enema coffee, which I gladly accepted. When I picked it up for use, however, I seriously wondered whether it was the proper strength. I have used enemas for many years and know pretty well what the coffee should look like. This solution seemed too weak to be considered "concentrate" for a dilution of 4 to 1. The lady "thought" that she used the recipe in the Handbook and that it was right. The caregiver must be sure that each enema contains the equivalent of 3 rounded tablespoons of coffee. (See A Cancer Therapy, p. 249.) If a concentrate is prepared, each portion MUST contain the 3 tablespoons of coffee. The coffee enema, too, is so very important that it is imperative that the mixture or solution is correct. Please check and re-check the preparation of the coffee concentrate.

5. Somewhat less important than the above four points: The patient enjoys some bread with his meals—which is quite acceptable. But it is also important to understand that the main requirements for nutrition are the salads, soup, potato, vegetables, and fruit. If all those foods have been consumed, it is all right for the patient to also have a slice of unsalted

rye bread. Bread should never be the main part of a meal. Unfortunately, in the last few months, we have had several patients who failed. I also discussed this problem with the most experienced Gerson Therapy doctors: Alicia Melendez and Luz Maria Bravo. Aside from the above, there are other problems we have run across. Let me state here that we (the Gerson doctors as well as myself when I talk to patients) have a serious problem. When we ask the patient about their compliance with the Gerson Therapy directives, even the above patient who made serious errors, will assure us that he is doing everything "perfectly." These patients don't realize what is wrong with their version of the Therapy. When we try to help, heal, and direct the patient on the Gerson Therapy, we rely on the various tools that we have specially created to give the patient and family every possible help and guidance: the food preparation video-tape and the recipe book in the Handbook; the four-hour workshop tape discussing in detail as much of the treatment as we can; and, most importantly, Dr. Gerson's book. At this point, I need to stress again that the patient must familiarize himself very thoroughly with this material and review it over and over again. One problem area that keeps coming up is the food preparation. Just boiling the vegetables and putting them on a plate is not good enough. The food preparation tape initiates the cook into various areas to make foods tasty. For example, cooked beets when peeled and sliced can be reheated a little with some freshly made applesauce and stirred. The vegetable then resembles Harvard beets. Or, the sliced beets can be dressed with onions, some green pepper strips, and vinegar with flax-seed oil dressing for a beet salad. During the summer months, these salads (also potato salad, string bean or butter bean salad, etc.) are very welcome, refreshing, and stimulating to the appetite. There are many suggested recipes in the back of the Handbook that, I am afraid, are being disregarded. As a result, we often get reports that the patients are weak, losing weight, and doing poorly. Almost always, it turns out that they have "cravings" for pizza, enchiladas, or some other greasy, salty, forbidden food. They are simply hungry because they are not eating well-prepared, healing, nutritious Gerson meals. Gerson meals have another advantage: if the patient (or family member for that matter) eats fresh, organic food, it is truly satisfying. We often get reports that the companions lose their cravings for sweets or heavy desserts. But the key to success is eating tasty food that is prepared with imagination and inspiration from the recipes provided. I must remind patients frequently that when they are on a nutritional therapy, they are on nothing if they don't eat! If patients eat properly, most will gain weight if they are emaciated. Those who are too heavy will lose weight on the same regimen. Fruits that are in season in the summer, such as cherries, apricots, peaches, nectarines, plums, pears, and grapes are especially valuable— they are high in the best nutrients: vitamins, potassium, and enzymes. Not far behind are apples that are available virtually all year round. Patients (unless they are diabetic or suffer from Candida) should always eat much fruit at night, first thing in the morning, and anytime between meals. One summer food presents a problem: corn. It is perfectly all right to eat fresh corn. The difficulty is that everybody loves corn and during the season is likely to eat it to the exclusion of other vegetables. That is a very bad idea. The vegetables should provide variety and a large selection of special healing chemicals (phytochemicals) and trace minerals. Eating mostly one vegetable is not acceptable and does not fulfill the purpose. Let the guiding spirit of the patient be: "I'll do the best possible to help my sick body heal," rather than "I'll see how little I can do and still get away with it." From *Gerson Healing Newsletter,* Vol. 14, No. 5 (Sep.-Oct. 1999).

Dr. Gerson spent many years collecting data on his patients with cancer and has come to the conclusion that a whole body concept was necessary in order for better outcomes in healing. He along with Dr. Issels has pioneered the whole-body concept, which I believe to be a powerful and effective therapy in cancer. Any individual deciding to implement this approach to healing their cancer must be completely resolved to follow it with no compromise. As you can see from the above newsletter excerpt, the Gerson approach requires total commitment. This program may not be for you. Before deciding to implement it, speak to individuals that are veterans of the program. You will get the good and the difficult aspects of the program.

ABO Serotype Diet

Another popular diet is the Blood Type Diet. (See *Eat Right for Your Type,* Dr. Peter D'Adamo. G.P. Putnam's Sons. ISBN 0-399-14255-X.) The basic philosophy of this diet is that your blood type reflects your internal chemistry. The metabolism and absorption of nutrients are different for each of the blood types. The four blood types are A, B, AB, and O. Each of the blood types has its beneficial foods and the foods that must be avoided. This diet is recommended for improving the quality of nutrition and for various health concerns, including cancer.

OTHER DIET RECOMMENDATIONS

Some individuals seem to do very well following food-combining and acid/alkaline diets. In addition, there is also the basic "rainbow of color" approach, which simply means a colorful variety of whole foods, juicing, and the macrobiotic way of eating. These will be described briefly.

Food Combining and Acid/Alkaline

The basic approach of this diet is to keep your proteins and starches away from each other. For example: having a protein like fish with vegetables instead of fish and potato or rice. It is OK to have pasta (starch) and vegetables. In this diet, melons and fruits should be eaten separately. Nuts and seeds are usually snack meals. The philosophy of this diet is to lessen the load on the digestive tract for better digestion and absorption of the food. I have noticed benefits from this dietary approach.

In this dietary approach, it is thought that the more alkaline the food, the healthier you will be. Advocates of this diet say that alkalinity equals longevity. There are foods that can make your body more acidic or alkaline. The majority of the foods that are alkaline are vegetables and some fruits. Meats, dairy, and some grains tend to produce more acid. The more acidic people are, the more likely they will develop cancer or a degenerative disease.

Colorful Foods As Medicine

The diet is the best place to begin fighting cancer. A variety of colorful foods from vegetable and fruit sources free from pesticides and organically cultivated and grown are recommended. There are many good reference sources for this on the Internet. I would recommend that your team of health providers include a nutritionist familiar with whole foods that can work along with you in designing the most effective plan.

Juicing

Juicing should be an essential part of cancer therapy. Juicing the yellow, green, orange, and purple pigment fruits and vegetables is very nutritious and immune enhancing.

However, juicing depends upon the tolerance of the individual. If you are really tired and fatigued, you may not have the energy to juice and a friend or relative may have to help you during such an important time in your life. Another important aspect of juicing is that the fruits and vegetables that are selected must be the highest grade in season as well as organic. All of the produce must be washed in an organic food wash before juicing.

An example of vegetables and fruits to be juiced include: apple, pear, blueberry, blackberry, apricot, kale, lemon, spinach, onion, garlic, mustard greens, carrot, asparagus, wheat grass, tomatoes, etc. You may want to experiment a bit and combine the compatible flavors. Remember that color and hearty flavor are the key ingredients that make up a healing juice. I have observed many cancer patients gain energy and some even had their cancers go into remission by maintaining a strict vegetarian diet and juicing. Another option is to add a protein powder to your juice to boost up the protein value.

Protein Powders and Medical Food Powders

Immunocal®: Immunocal is a whey-based protein powder isolate that has powerful immune-modulating properties. It is used extensively in cancer to maintain nutritional health and to enhance immune health while a patient is receiving cancer treatment. Immunocal maintains a healthier immune system by sustaining levels of glutathione in the lymphocytes. Glutathione helps to support the proper functioning of your immune system.

- Your body's natural immune activity involving unimpeded multiplication of lymphocytes and antibody production requires maintenance of normal levels of glutathione inside the lymphocytes.

- Glutathione plays a central, protective role against the damaging effects of pollutants and free radicals.

- Without glutathione, other important antioxidants, such as vitamins C and E, cannot adequately do their job.

- The second major function of glutathione consists of the body's natural detoxification of foreign chemical compounds.

There are many patients who have benefited from the use of Immunocal, and I recommend it. However, if there is an allergy or sensitivity to whey, then I would find another alternative. For further information on Immunocal, you may search their web site at http://www.immunocal.com

UltraBalance medical food powders: Another quality product available in cancer treatment is the UltraBalance Medical Food Powders. I have utilized this product and incorporated it into the diet and treatment plan for my patients. UltraBalance Medical Foods are designed to nutritionally support patients with food sensitivities during detoxification and gastrointestinal support programs for general nutrition and during weight loss or weight maintenance. In cancer treatment, it is essential to maintain adequate nutritional intake. I highly recommend this as part of the cancer treatment program. For further information, contact www.ultrabalance.com

NUTRITIONAL GLANDULAR SUPPORT

A cancer treatment program that doesn't include support for the glands is not complete. Remember, cancer affects every organ, gland, and system. The glandular system includes the pituitary gland, thyroid gland, adrenal glands, and reproductive glands. All of these glands work together to keep hormone balance. Some cancers may directly involve these glands, making nutritional support imperative. Some nutritional supports to consider:

- Adrenal support formula (should include adrenal gland, pantothenic acid, panax ginseng, licorice root, zinc, and other supportive B vitamins): Some good formula recommendations are Cortrex (Thorne Research) and Adrenoplex (Priority One). Before beginning any of these formulas, consult your doctor. The adrenal glands are crucial in regulating your body's response to stress and balanced replacement may be essential to keep strong adrenals.

- Thyroid support formula (should include thyroid gland, L-tyrosine, and thyroid balancing herbs): Some good formula recommendations are Spectra 303-T (NF Formulations) and Thyrotropic PMG (Standard Process Labs). Before beginning any of these formulas, consult your doctor. It is important to periodically monitor the thyroid, and it may be necessary to correct low thyroid output with Levoxyl and/ or Cytomel, which are both synthetic hormones. It is not uncommon to have diminished thyroid output during chemotherapy and radiation therapy.

- Other supportive nutrients for better glandular support include free-form amino acids, CoQ10, panax ginseng, vitamin B12, folic acid, and DHEA.

Chapter 12

Herbal Therapies and Cancer Treatment

Cancer studies indicate that cancer develops when the body's immune system is weakened; therefore, a strengthened immune system is crucial in the fight against cancer. Plant medicines, when taken appropriately, can offer immune-strengthening, tumor-fighting, hormone-balancing, nutritive, and cleansing properties.

Many herbal therapies focus on restoring health to the body's immune system so the body can work to fight against cancer. Various herbs are being carefully studied to determine their beneficial use, not only in fighting cancer, but also in curing the disease. When shopping for quality herbal medicine be sure that they are certified organically grown and single herbs or compatible formulations

ANTICANCER EFFECTS OF PHYTONUTRIENTS

Plant medicines have a number of valuable characteristics. We will discuss some of these plant medicines used in cancer treatment in some detail as we move along. However, generally speaking, I would like to illustrate for you below a table of phytonutrients and their action.

Phytonutrient	Source	Action
Carotenes	• Dark-colored fruits and vegetables	• Antioxidants • Immune modulating
Coumarin	• Citrus fruits, carrots	• Anti-tumor • Immune modulating • Antioxidant
Flavonoids	• Fruits, citrus fruits, tomatoes	• Antioxidant • Anti-tumor • Immune-modulating
Isoflavinoids	• Soy and legumes	• Estrogen receptor modifier
Lignans	• Flax seed flax oil, grains, nuts, and seeds	• Antioxidant • Hormone receptor modulator
Limonoids	• Citrus fruits	• Detoxification • Decreases carcinogenic activity
Polyphenols	• Green tea, red wine, chocolate	• Antioxidant • Decreases carcinogenic activity • Hormone receptor modulator
Sterols	• Soy, nuts, and seeds	• Decreases carcinogenic activity • Hormone receptor modulator
Sulfur-containing nutrients (Dithiolthiones, Thiocyanates, Glucosinolates)	• Cabbage, broccoli, brussel sprouts, kale	• Detoxification • Decreases carcinogenic activity

HERBS USED IN CANCER THERAPY

The pharmaceutical drugs found in nature contain significant healing powers. The following list of natural herbs provides a description of the herb, active ingredients, common uses, dosing, adverse reactions, and contraindications.

Warning: Natural does not always mean safe. Recommended therapies are only advised under the supervision of your health care provider.

Aloe Vera

This plant's origin is Africa. The parts of the plant used are its leaves and roots. The plant produces a gel substance that contains many active compounds. Aloe had been used historically for the treatment of constipation. The root of the plant was used for intestinal colic. Aloe has also been used in India to treat intestinal infections.

> **Active ingredients:** The compounds aloe contains include acemannan, anthrone-10- C-glykosyls, including aloin A, aloin B, 7-hydroxyaloins and 1, 8-dihydroxyanthraquinones, including aloe-emodin. Aloe also contains flavonoids and resins.

> **Uses in cancer therapy:** Aloe gel can be beneficial in stimulating immunity. In animal studies, a water-soluble compound was found in aloe vera known as acemannan. This compound is a potent immune stimulant and anti-tumor agent.

> **Dosing:** Criteria for therapeutic dosing has not been established for humans. For constipation, a single dose of 50–200 mg should be taken each day for a maximum of ten days. Topical application of a stabilized gel may be used for minor burns. For more serious burns, a health professional must be contacted before

application is made. Internal use of the gel is at 30 ml three times daily.

Adverse reactions: There have been some reports of allergic reactions to aloe, but it is rare. If used as a laxative, aloe must not be used for more than ten consecutive days. Chronic use of aloe can lead to potassium deficiency, especially when used with licorice, thiazide diuretics, and steroids. The actions of cardiac and antiarhythmic drugs can be affected by the use of aloe.

Contraindications: Aloe should not be used in cases of intestinal obstruction and acutely inflamed intestinal diseases (ulcerative colitis, Crohn's disease), appendicitis, and abdominal pain of unknown origin. Aloe should not be used in pregnancy and in children under twelve years of age.

Amygdalin

Amygdalin is also known as Laetrile, or vitamin B17. This substance is concentrated in kernels of apricots. Amygdalin has been used in China for centuries. It has demonstrated strong cancer-fighting potential in general. Amygdalin is given both orally and intravenously. There is much controversy over its use and benefits in cancer treatment. Dosing depends upon the type of cancer.

Arabinogalactans (Larix)

Larix, known as an immune enhancer, is a sweet-tasting powder derived from the Western Larch tree (*Larix occidentalis*). Dr. Peter D'Adamo identified and developed Larix from a paper by-product. The immune related effects of Larix powder include:

- stimulation of NK cells activity

- stimulation of macrophage activity

- enhanced tumor cell-killing due to increased immune response

- stimulation

Dosing is usually one teaspoon twice daily. Larix is available from Eclectic Institute at 1.800.332.4372.

Artemesia extract

Artemesia is a plant medicine that has shown some promise in the treatment of breast and prostate cancer. Two researchers at the University of Washington Medical School are evaluating Artemesia. It is said that the active constituents arrest cancer cells and enhance cytokine activity. One of the most recent studies reveal that the action of Artemesia is enhanced by the use of Vitamin C. There is also a connection between high iron and cancer progression. Artemesia's effects involve serum and tissue levels of iron but the connection is not clearly understood at this time. I have used this herb in my practice on several cases with excellent results. In the cases I have treated with Artemesia clinical improvement has resulted. Total remission of cancer has been achieved in four cases currently. See Appendix 5 for further information on Artemesia therapy.

Astragalus (Astragalus Membranaceus)

This plant's origin is China. The main part of the plant used is its root, which is aged four to seven years before use. In cancer therapy, this botanical is very useful for enhancing immune response and in chemotherapy support.

- Active ingredients: Astragalus contains flavonoids, polysaccharides, triterpene glycosides (e.g., astraglycosides I–VII), amino acids, and trace minerals. Astragalus has action on the white blood cells and is used in cancer treatment to restore counts toward the reference range.

- Uses: Traditional Chinese medicine uses this herb for night sweats, fatigue, loss of appetite, weakness, and diarrhea. Empirical medicine has used this herb for the common cold, sore throat, and general immune modulating.

- Dosage: The recommended dosing for Astragalus is 500 mg, two to three capsules, three times daily or 3–5 ml three times daily. There are no negative side effects known when used as recommended.

Cat's claw (Uncaria guianensis; Uncaria tomentosa)

Cat's claw, or *uña de gato*, as it is also called, has piqued many people's interest lately. First, because it comes from remote and exotic rain forests, and second, because it is believed to act on the immune system. Both of the species referred to as cat's claw are climbing woody vines (lianas) in the Amazon Rain Forest. The name refers to the small sharp spines on the stem, near the leaf, curved back like a cat's claw. *U. guianensis* has been used by native people in South America to treat intestinal problems and to heal wounds.

The bark is used by different tribes for different purposes: some find it an effective contraceptive and others use it to treat gonorrhea. This plant is widely used to relieve the pain of rheumatism and to reduce inflammation, as well as for dysentery and ulcers. This species of cat's claw is preferred in the European market. *U. tomentosa*, from the Peruvian headwaters of the Amazon, is often used for arthritis, ulcers, and other intestinal problems. In addition, it is prized as a general tonic for its "life-giving" properties and is used for certain skin diseases. The North American marketplace provides the major commercial outlet for this species. The bark is the part of the plant generally used for medicinal purposes. The use of this herb in cancer treatment is becoming more prominent, demonstrating some anti-tumor characteristics and immune-enhancing properties.

- Active ingredients: Research on the constituents of uña de gato was begun only a few decades ago. Both species appear to contain alkaloids. *U. tomentosa* also contains quinovic acid glycosides and some novel triterpenes.

- Uses: Traditional use by Amazonian tribes includes the treatment of a number of digestive disorders. Uña de gato is sometimes promoted in the United States to treat problems such as hemorrhoids, gastritis, colitis, ulcers, diverticulitis, and leaky bowel. These applications appear to be based more on reports of folk medicine from the Amazon than on clinical or animal studies. In the test tube, most of the alkaloids of *U. tomentosa* can be shown to activate immune-system cells. Several quinovic acid glycosides are active against various viruses in the laboratory. Many of these compounds also counteract inflammation caused experimentally in rat-paw tests. One important alkaloid lowers blood pressure, relaxes and dilates peripheral blood vessels, slows heart rate, and lowers cholesterol. Another acts as a diuretic. The immune-stimulating effects of *U. tomentosa* have attracted attention for the possibility that the herb might be useful against cancer.

- Dosage: One gram of root bark to one cup of boiling water, steeped for ten minutes. After cooling and straining, one cup is drunk two-three times per day. In tincture form, 1–2 ml, two times per day. In standardized extract, between 20–60 mg per day.

- Contraindications: Pregnant women should not take cat's claw because its safety and mode of action have been inadequately studied.

- Adverse effects: No serious reactions have been reported in the literature.

- Possible interactions: No interactions with other drugs or herbs have been reported in the literature. Because of the limited information available, it seems prudent not to combine *U. tomentosa* with other herbs or drugs that affect the immune system, such as cortisone-like drugs or cyclosporine.

Echinacea

Echinacea is the name of a genus of native North American plants with reddish or purplish flowers. There are nine species, but only three of them *(E. angustifolia, E. pallida, E. purpurea)* are used as botanical medicines. Gardeners may recognize Echinacea as the purple coneflower. Many Native American tribes, to treat snakebite and many other ailments, used Echinacea traditionally, and settlers learned of its properties from the Indians. Most of the research on the chemistry and pharmacology of these plants has been conducted in Europe, where, until fairly recently, Echinacea was a much more popular herb than in the United States. The current enthusiasm for Echinacea derives from research suggesting that it can stimulate the immune system and help fight off viral infections, such as colds or influenza. In this country, Echinacea is available primarily as a tincture (alcohol-based extract) or as capsules of dried leaves and stems collected when the plant is in flower. There are also standardized extracts of Echinacea available.

- Active ingredients: The three species are not interchangeable, although they may sometimes be confused with one another. Each may have a different balance of active compounds. Of course, the roots also differ from the aboveground parts of the plant, though both are utilized medicinally. The chemistry of Echinacea is complex, and no single ingredient has been identified as primarily responsible for the therapeutic activity. A caffeic acid glycoside, echinacoside, makes up approximately 0.1% of the leaves and stems, which also contain cichoric acid.

Fresh Echinacea or its juice contains a volatile sub-stance not found in the dried plant material. The roots of *E. angustifolia* contain chemicals called alkamides.

- Uses: Echinacea has become extremely popular for the treatment of colds, influenza, and other respira-tory tract infections. Although the herb does not seem to kill viruses directly, it is believed to stimu-late or modulate the immune system, allowing the host to fight off infection. In one European study, people taking Echinacea recovered from their colds four days earlier than those taking a placebo. Both the root of *E. pallida* and the above ground parts of *E. purpurea* are used in Europe for this purpose. It is usually given just at the first appearance of symp-toms, rather than taken daily as a preventive.

- One study of three hundred people (in three groups, taking *E. purpurea, E. angustifolia,* or a placebo) over twelve weeks was not able to demonstrate a signifi-cant advantage of the botanical medicines over the placebo. The authors hypothesize that Echinacea might reduce the rate of infection by 10% to 20%, undetectable at that sample size. The herb is given orally or by injection in Germany for other infec-tions as well, including prostatitis and urinary tract infections.

- Test tube and animal research has shown that Echinacea extracts have significant anti-inflamma-tory activity. When applied to the skin, the extract is almost as effective as a potent anti-inflammatory drug, indomethacin, used topically. Topically, the extracts have been used to help hasten the healing of stubborn wounds, eczema, psoriasis, and herpes simplex. To maximize the benefit of the herb, it

211

should be given together with a multiple vitamin. (In Australia, a formulation that includes Echinacea, vitamin A, vitamin C, vitamin E, zinc, and garlic is prescribed at the first sign of viral respiratory infection.) Preliminary studies suggest that it may be of some use in treating certain cancers. Much more research is needed on this potential application.

- Dosage: When fresh-squeezed juice is used, the dose is 6 to 9 ml, or approximately one and one-half teaspoons (= 7.5 ml). Other oral formulations should supply the equivalent of 900 mg of the herb daily. One study indicated that short-term use could boost cell-mediated immunity, but that repeated use over a period of weeks reduced the immune response. This interpretation of the results has been questioned, but most authorities suggest six to eight weeks as the maximum time to take Echinacea preparations. One study using the fresh juice of *E. purpurea* showed no problems for people taking it for up to twelve weeks. The herb should be stored away from light to maintain potency.

- Special precautions: Many authorities warn against using Echinacea for people with autoimmune diseases, multiple sclerosis, or other serious conditions, such as tuberculosis, AIDS, or leukemia. These precautions appear to rest on theoretical grounds and are not universally accepted, but we believe it is prudent to respect them.

- Adverse reactions: Side effects have rarely been reported with the use of Echinacea. In a recent study of Echinacea extracts for the prevention of colds, 18% of the patients taking *E. angustifolia,* 10% of those taking *E. purpurea,* and 11% of those on placebo experienced side effects. The researchers did not specify what reactions occurred but reported that they were not serious and did not require treatment. Echinacea has an unpleasant aftertaste.

- Possible interactions: Interactions of Echinacea with other medications are based on theoretical concerns. Some of the alkaloids found in Echinacea are similar to plant chemicals that can be damaging to the liver. Thus, some doctors suggest that Echinacea should not be used with other drugs that can have negative effects on the liver, such as Nizoral, methotrexate, Cordarone, or anabolic steroids. One reference notes that flavonoids found in E. *purpurea* affect the enzyme (CYP 3A4) responsible for metabolizing many common drugs. This is the same enzyme affected by grapefruit, but we do not know if the effect would be clinically important. If it were, medications as varied as cyclosporine, Plendil, Procardia, Sular, Propulsid, Hismanal, Mevacor, Zocor, Tegretol, or Viagra could reach higher levels in the body. Coumadin might also be affected. Monitoring drug response is important.

Essiac Herbs

Essiac, a harmless herbal tea, was used by Canadian nurse Rene Caisse to successfully treat thousands of cancer patients from the 1920s until her death in 1978 at the age of 90. Refusing payment for her services, instead accepting only voluntary contributions, the Bracebridge, Ontario, nurse brought remissions to hundreds of documented cases, many abandoned as "hopeless" or "terminal" by orthodox medicine. She aided countless more in prolonging life and relieving pain. Caisse obtained remarkable results against a wide variety of cancers, treating persons by administering Essiac through hypodermic injection or oral ingestion. The following benefits may result from the use of Essiac:

- prevent build-up of excess fatty deposits in artery walls, heart, kidney tubules, and liver;

- regulate cholesterol levels by transforming sugar and fat into energy;

- halt diarrhea, check internal hemorrhaging, and overcome constipation;

- counteract the detrimental effects of aluminum, lead, and mercury poisoning;

- strengthen and tighten muscles, organs, and tissues;

- make bones, joints, ligaments, lungs, and membranes strong and flexible, more durable, and less vulnerable to stress;

- nourish and stimulate the brain and nervous system;

- promote the absorption of fluids in the tissues;

- remove toxic accumulation in the fat, lymph, bone marrow, bladder, and alimentary canal;

- neutralize acids, absorb toxins in bowel, and help to eliminate both;

- relieve the liver of its burden of detoxification by converting fatty toxins into water-soluble substances that can be easily eliminated through the kidneys;

- reduce, perhaps eliminate, heavy metal deposits in tissues, especially those surrounding the joints, to relieve inflammation and stiffness;

- improve the functions of the pancreas and spleen by increasing the effectiveness of insulin;

- increase red cell production;

- increase the body's ability to utilize oxygen by raising the oxygen level in tissue cells;

- maintain the balance between potassium and sodium within the body so the fluid inside and outside each cell is regulated. In this way, cells are nourished with nutrients and are cleansed;

- protect against toxins entering the brain;

- protect the body against radiation and X-rays;

- relieve pain, increase the appetite, and provide more energy with a sense of well-being;

- speed up wound healing by regenerating the damaged area;

- increase the production of antibodies like lymphocytes in the thymus gland, defenders of our immune system;

- inhibit and possibly destroy benign growths and tumors.

Essiac Herbs

- Burdock Root (*Arctium lappa*)
- Sheep Sorrel (*Rumex acetosella*)
- Turkey Rhubarb Root (*Rheum palmatum*)
- Slippery Elm Bark (ulmus fulva)

The herbs can be made into a tea, powdered extract, and tincture.

Garlic

Garlic is valued in many parts of the world for its pungent aroma and flavor. It is possible that garlic's biological activity and popularity in Mediterranean diet cuisine contribute to the healthful effects of the "Mediterranean diet." Garlic was used in the nineteenth century for tuberculosis and into World War

II for disinfecting battlefield wounds. It is frequently used in an attempt to ward off or treat the common colds. The herb is available in many forms, including fresh bulbs, oil-based extracts, dried powder, and steam-distilled extracts. To maximize the anti-cancer activity of fresh garlic in cooking, crush or mince it at least ten minutes before heating.

> **Active ingredients:** Sulfur compounds give garlic its characteristic pungent aroma and probably account for some of the flavor. They also appear to be responsible for most of the medicinal properties of this herb, although the trace minerals germanium and selenium may also play a role. An inert compound, alliin, is converted to allicin once the clove is cut or crushed. In Europe, standardized extracts of garlic are supposed to contain at least 0.45% allicin, a compound that breaks down into most of the active components, such as ajoene. Chemical analysis of garlic products shows that concentrations of sulfur compounds vary enormously.

> Uses: Garlic is widely used for its cardiovascular benefits, although the results of two American trials on its ability to lower cholesterol were disappointing. An analysis of twenty-six other studies showed that cholesterol was reduced, on the average, by approximately 10%. In some studies, dangerous LDL cholesterol dropped by 16%, while other research has shown increases in beneficial HDL with long-term use. Although the cholesterol-lowering power of garlic appears modest, the herb is reported to reduce oxidation of LDL and seems to have other cardio-protective effects. Several garlic-derived chemicals can help slow blood clotting by keeping blood platelets from clumping together. In addition, garlic helps to break up or prevent blood clots through fibrinolytic action. Since many heart attacks

and strokes are believed to be caused by spontaneous clots in blood vessels, these anticoagulant actions could be very helpful. Garlic may also lower blood pressure, but it is less effective in this respect than are medicines. It is helpful, however, in keeping blood vessels to the heart flexible in older people.

One of the most intriguing possibilities for garlic is that regular ingestion may help prevent cancer. Studies in China, comparing people in one region where garlic is commonly eaten (20 grams, or approximately seven cloves a day, on average) with those in another region where daily consumption is less than half a clove, found the garlic eaters were much less likely to suffer stomach cancer. Other studies have indicated that people who eat garlic more often seem less susceptible to stomach or colon cancer. Animal research confirms that garlic has the potential to improve resistance to tumors, and test-tube research shows that garlic can interfere with some cancer-causing chemicals.

Adverse effects: In rats, high doses of garlic led to weight loss and damage to the stomach lining. Humans taking garlic oil at a dose equivalent to twenty cloves daily for three months did not report problems. Most people appear to tolerate garlic well, but some individuals experience digestive distress. People who handle garlic products occasionally develop a skin reaction on exposure (contact dermatitis). Ingesting fresh garlic and most extracts results in a characteristic breath odor. This has been linked to the active sulfur-containing compounds. Parsley is recommended as a home remedy for garlic breath.

Possible interactions: Although there are no studies of interactions, in theory, garlic could increase the risk of bleeding in people taking anticoagulants, such as

Coumadin, aspirin, Plavix, or Ticlid. There is also a possibility that this herb could interact with drugs such as DiaBeta or Glucotrol that lower blood sugar. Careful monitoring is suggested for anyone combining garlic products with such prescription drugs.

Garlic appears to inhibit an enzyme called CYP 2E1. In most cases, this interference is welcome, since this enzyme can make carcinogens more dangerous. But CYP 2E1 is also involved in the metabolism of acetaminophen (Panadol, Tylenol, etc.) and a muscle relaxant called chlorzoxazone (Parafon Forte). These drugs could possibly linger longer in people who are taking or eating garlic.

Graviola

Graviola is a plant medicine that has demonstrated some positive results in the treatment of cancer. It is an evergreen that grows in South and North America in warmer climates. In an 1976 plant screening program by the National Cancer Institute, the leaves and stem of Graviola showed active cytotoxicity against cancer cells and researchers have been following up on this research ever since. It is said that this plant has potent anti-tumor properties. Extensive studies have been achieved at Purdue University. Further research is necessary to evaluate its safety in cancer therapy.

Green Tea

Green tea extract is used in cancer primarily to reduce risk and enhance immune function. It contains many vitamins and minerals as well as some other important ingredients listed below.

> **Active ingredients:** The methylxanthine alkaloids, caffeine, theophylline, and theobromine, comprise between 1 and 5% of tea. These compounds have

similar but not identical actions; caffeine is usually the dominant one. Depending on the variety of tea and the way it was prepared, a cup (a proper six-ounce teacup) may contain from 10 to 50 mg of caffeine. Low doses of caffeine may actually slow heart rate slightly, while higher doses can speed heart rate or even contribute to mild rhythm abnormalities. Green tea, like black tea, is rich in tannins. Tannic acids make up 9% to 20% of the leaves. Flavonoids, including apigenin, kaempferol, myricetin, and quercetin, have also been identified but at low concentrations. Some flavonoids unique to black tea are theaflavins, theasinensins, thearubigens, and theacitrins. Another set of flavonoids has been intensively studied recently. These polyphenols (catechins) are not vitamins, but they seem to have strong antioxidant properties. Epigallocatechin-3-gallate (EGCG), in particular, has been identified as capable of protecting experimental animals from radiation damage and possibly reducing the risk of cancer.

Uses: Current interest in green tea in the United States has focused mainly on its cancer-preventive properties rather than on its flavor, which may be an acquired taste. Japanese researchers were the first to report that people living in an area where green tea was an important crop were only half or even a fifth as likely to develop cancer as those in an area that did not grow tea. There seems to be an inverse relationship between drinking tea and developing cancer of the digestive tract or urinary system. One recent epidemiological study in Japan showed that men who drank ten or more cups of green tea daily had a significantly lower risk of lung, liver, colon, or stomach cancer.

EGCG seems to be responsible in large measure for inhibiting the growth of cancer cells and mopping up free radicals that can damage healthy cells. It also appears to work on the heterocyclic amines that form when meat, poultry, or fish is grilled and keeps them from initiating cancerous changes. One Chinese study suggests that green tea can counteract the cancer-promoting effects of female hormones on breast tissue. Further research on this is needed. The polyphenols in green tea are thought to be responsible for its chemo-preventive activity. Curcumin seems to act synergistically with green tea in preventing mutations and tumor development.

EGCG also has antibacterial and antiviral activity and stimulates the immune system to produce interleukin-1 and tumor necrosis factor. These and possibly other actions may explain the capacity of EGCG to reduce periodontitis; and this, in turn, may explain how green tea helps minimize bad breath. Prospective trials have not shown that tea lowers blood lipids. Because tea discourages oxidation of low-density lipoprotein, however, it may help protect against atherosclerosis. Both green tea and Earl Grey counteracted platelet clumping and prevented coronary blood clots in a dog experiment, but scientists have not been able to demonstrate any anti-platelet effect in humans. Topical application of EGCG from green tea in animal experiments stopped the development of skin cancer after exposure to a carcinogenic chemical. Polyphenols from green tea can also protect skin from ultraviolet radiation (UV-B) damage, acting essentially as a natural sunscreen.

Dose: Approximately 2 g of tea is used with 250 ml of boiling water. Large doses of green tea, up to nine or ten cups daily, were associated with cardiovascular benefit in the early epidemiological studies. These results have not been confirmed. Daily use of green tea by much of the population in China and Japan suggests that no strict time limits on administration need be observed.

Special precautions: High doses of caffeine have been linked to infertility and birth defects. Large amounts of green tea are, therefore, not recommended for pregnant women or those attempting to conceive. Caffeine is detectable in breast milk after the mother consumes a caffeine-containing beverage. The diuretic effects of caffeine and theophylline may put a strain on kidneys with pre-existing problems. People with ulcers, heart rhythm problems, and clinical anxiety disorders should minimize their intake of caffeine.

Adverse effects: People who drink excessive amounts of green tea may get too much caffeine. High concentrations of caffeine (hard to achieve with moderate green tea intake) can result in rapid heart rate or altered heart rhythm (PVC), excess fluid elimination, jitteriness, and insomnia. Chronic use of caffeine can lead to symptoms of headache, sluggishness, and irritability upon withdrawal. Withdrawal has been reported in people who stop drinking as little as two or three cups of coffee daily and, therefore, might be anticipated in people who suddenly stop drinking many cups of green tea (five or six daily).

Possible interactions: The tannins in tea can interfere with the absorption of non-heme iron (iron supplements, for example) taken at the same time. Milk added to black tea can reduce the binding capacity of tannins. (Milk is rarely, if ever, added to green tea.) Caffeine (65 mg) can increase the analgesic effects of aspirin or acetaminophen. Antibiotics, such as Cipro, Noroxin, or Penetrex, and the ulcer drug Tagamet (cimetidine), can increase the stimulant effects of caffeine. Combining tea with a medication containing theophylline or caffeine could result in too much caffeine and cause nervousness or insomnia.

Hoxsey Formula

In the early 1900s, Harry Hoxsey developed an herbal formula that he believed was effective for the treatment of cancer. It consists of two remedies: one to be used externally; the other, internally. The external mixture is said to be selectively destructive of cancerous tissue and consists of a red paste—containing antimony trisulfide, zinc chloride, and bloodroot—and a yellow powder—containing arsenic sulfide, sulfur, and talc. The internal mixture is a liquid containing licorice, red clover, burdock root, stillingia root, barberry, cascara, prickly ash bark, buckthorn bark, and potassium iodide. This mixture is considered to be cathartic/cleansing, or immune-boosting. Hoxsey felt that his therapy normalized and balanced the body's chemistry makeup, allowing it to essentially create a self-healing environment in which the immune system is strengthened and tumors are caused to die. The treatment is available in Tijuana, Mexico.

> **Dosage:** The dose of the therapy varies depending on the specific needs of each patient and whether the cancer is internal or on the skin. The preparation is used either directly on the skin or drunk as a tonic. Patients are encouraged to *avoid* pork, vinegar, tomatoes, carbonated drinks, and alcohol, and to *use* immune stimulants, yeast tablets, vitamin C, calcium, laxatives, and antiseptic washes as well as adopt a positive mental outlook while taking the Hoxsey treatment.

Adverse reactions: Some of the ingredients in the Hoxsey formula can cause side effects. For instance, buckthorn bark can cause nausea, vomiting, and diarrhea if taken in large quantities. Cascara can cause diarrhea. Barberry root administered to rabbits (dose unspecified) caused swelling of the kidney and cardiotoxicity. Diarrhea can lead to dehydration and electrolyte imbalance.

Iscador (Mistletoe Extract)

Iscador is a remedy used by European physicians. It is the trade name for the herb mistletoe. In animal experiments, Iscador has been found to kill cancer cells, stimulate the immune system, and inhibit tumor formation. Iscador is available from Waleda at 1.800.241.1030. Extreme caution should be used when using this herb and always under the supervision of your physician that specializes in integrative medicine.

Milk Thistle (Silybum marianum)

This herb is grown in varied places. You may find it along roadsides and grown wild in different climates. The seeds of the dried flower are used. In cancer, this herb is primarily used in chemotherapy support. It enhances liver detoxification and supports the growth of healthy liver cells.

Uses: Milk thistle has been used for hundreds of years. It was prescribed in liver and gallbladder conditions often. It was used in the treatment of jaundice. This herb is an all-around safe and effective medicine. Milk thistle contains a bioflavonoid known as silymarin. Silymarin is made up of three constituents: silibinin, silidianin, and silicristin. The action of silibinin is responsible for medicinal benefits of silymarin. Milk thistle protects liver cells against toxins and is known to cause the healthy growth of new liver cells.

Dosage: Milk thistle is relatively safe and devoid of any side effects. In liver disease, it is recommended 400–1,000 mg of milk thistle be given. If you prefer to use it in the form of food, 12–15 grams of seeds can be ground. However, this by no means will have a therapeutic effect on the liver.

Adverse reactions: Milk thistle is free from any side effects and can be used in a wide range of health conditions. Some may notice a mild laxative effect with using this herb.

Contraindications and possible interactions: None currently known.

Mushroom Extract and PSK/PSP

Shiitake and maitake mushroom extracts and isolates have been used in a variety of cancers. Maitake mushroom extracts demonstrate more powerful anti-tumor properties. Maitake has inhibiting effects on carcinogenesis (development of cancer) and metastasis (the spread of cancer). Shiitake is also used in cancer, but it is not as strong of an anticancer variety.

Pau d'arco (*Tabebuia impetiginosa; Tabebuia avellanedae*)

Pau d'arco, known as *lapacho colorado* in Argentina and Paraguay and as *ipe roxo* in Brazil, is a good example of the lure of the exotic. This South American native has been used medicinally by several indigenous groups. There are several species of *Tabebuia*, and most appear to be broad-leaved evergreen trees with very hard wood that resists decay. It may be difficult to determine precisely which species is being sold as pau d'arco tea. Pau d'arco has a reputation for having been used by the Incas, although it is not native to the high Andes.

Uses: It is said to be useful against cancer, diabetes, rheumatism, and ulcers, as well as several other ailments. The part of the tree used is the inner bark, and the preparation made from it is sometimes termed *taheebo*. Pau d'arco, or taheebo, contains a number of quinone compounds, including the naphthoquinone lapachol and the anthraquinone tabebuin. These and related compounds are assumed to be the active ingredients. Lapachol has antibacterial activity, and a related compound fights off fungus and yeast. Lapachol has demonstrated activity against malaria, a property that would certainly be useful for people in the areas where Tabebuia species grow wild.

Test-tube and animal research in the 1950s and 1960s indicated that taheebo extract and lapachol could slow the growth of certain tumors. In human trials, it was difficult to attain therapeutically active levels of lapachol with oral administration, and when levels did get high enough, most people suffered serious adverse effects, such as nausea and vomiting. Taheebo extract has anti-inflammatory activity, at least in rats. Researchers have also found that it helps animals resist ulcers. In laboratory studies on human blood cells, lapachol had immunosuppressant effects at higher doses and immunostimulant activity at low doses.

Dosage: Standard dose has not been determined. Recommended 500 mg daily.

Contraindications: Pregnant women should not take taheebo internally, because there is no evidence of its safety, and it can provoke adverse reactions. Pau d'arco should be discontinued before surgery because of the danger of excessive bleeding. Studies of pau d'arco in humans have noted reactions, such as severe nausea, vomiting, diarrhea, dizziness, anemia, and bleeding. Administering vitamin K will stop the bleeding. The fact that taheebo causes vitamin K-reversible bleeding strongly suggests that it would interact with anticoagulants, such as Coumadin, to increase the danger of hemorrhage.

Pectin

Pectin has demonstrated some useful effects in stopping the spread of cancer in animal studies. It is a fiber derived from citrus and tolerated well by the body. Pectin is known to increase immune activity against cancer cells. It comes as a powder and can be taken in juice or water. For cancers that have spread to other sites, it is important to include this in the cancer treatment regimen.

PC-Spes

This formulation blends together eight herbs for use in the treatment of prostate cancer. It is also demonstrating some benefits in other forms of cancer, including sarcoma and breast cancer, although this formulation is not used primarily in these cancers. The use of PC-SPES in prostate cancer has demonstrated hopeful results. In a study conducted by the University of California at San Francisco, seventy participants had 100% decline in their PSA. PC-SPES demonstrates the following activities:

1. immune-stimulating

2. anti-tumor

3. anti-viral

4. anti-inflammatory

5. decreased bioavailability of testosterone

Herbs in PC-SPES:

- Isatis indigotica (da qing ye)

- Glycyrrhiza glabra and Gycyrrhiza uralensis (gancao), also known as licorice root

- Panax ginseng (san qi)

- Ganoderma lucidum (ling zhi)

- Scutellaria baicalensis (huang qin)

- Dendranthema (chrysanthemum)

- Rabdosia rebescens

- Saw palmetto (serenoa repens)

Each of these herbs works together in enhancing immune action, inducing apoptosis (programmed cancer cell death), working against the tumor, increasing NK cell activity, modulating hormonal balance, and maintaining homeostasis (system balance). For further information on PC SPES consult the following references:

- *The Best Options for Diagnosing and Treating Prostate Cancer* by James Lewis Jr., Ph.D. ISBN 1-883257-042.

- *The Herbal Remedy for Prostate Cancer* by James Lewis Jr., Ph.D. ISBN 1-883257-02-6.

- Other traditional Chinese herbs can be referenced in the book *Cancer and Natural Medicine*. This book is an excellent resource for identifying potentially useful herbs in cancer treatment. Written by John Boik. Oregon Medical Press. ISBN 0-9648280-0-6.

Adverse reactions:

- allergy to formulation

- blood clot formation in legs and/or lungs

- changes in urine flow

- decreased ability to maintain erection

- decreased sexual desire

- diarrhea

- leg cramps and/or muscle cramping

There is much controversy over the use of PC SPES in prostate cancer because the herbs cannot deliver a consistent dose of the active agents. The FDA ordered PC SPES off of the market because of its undetermined amount of a drug named Coumadin (Warfarin) that is used as a potent blood thinner. I understand that the protection of the public from harm should be the highest order of importance. The FDA determined that this is unsafe for the public because of possible negative reactions is valid. However, there is always some issue taken when an agent is an effective treatment. Effective treatments automatically are often under scrutiny (i.e. Hydrazine controversy). If such measures were used with pharmaceutical drugs, countless Americans could have been protected from very serious drug reactions over the last several decades.

My recommendation is that the combination herbs in PC-SPES be used with caution and under the supervision of a physician specializing in natural medicine. There is a vast amount of information on PC-SPES on the Internet. It is best to consult your physician if considering this formulation.

TRADITIONAL CHINESE HERBS

There are many traditional Chinese herbs that are currently used in the treatment of cancer. Many have demonstrated potential. However, there must be continued medical study to determine safety and effectiveness of the herbs. Traditional Chinese herbs are used in a different way than what we are familiar with here in America. For more information, see the section on Chinese tradition in medical treatment.

Fu Zhen Therapy

Used in hospitals in China for the treatment of cancer. This therapy increases the activity of nonspecific immune cells. The following herbs are used in this treatment: ginseng, ligustrum, astragalus, codonopsis, astracylodes, and ganoderma. The aim of therapy is to restore energy, enhance digestion, and strengthen the immune system.

Liu Wei Di Huang

Used primarily in lung cancer. It is also known as the Six-Flavor Tea. This Chinese formulation is said to have anti-tumor effects.

Jian Pi Yi Qi Li Shui (Polyporus umbellatus)

This herb is used to reduce the risk of injury to the kidneys while undergoing chemotherapy. It also exhibits anti-tumor effects by stimulating immune activity around tumor sites.

● ●

Chapter 13

Common Alternative Treatment Options

When pursuing a therapy that you are unfamiliar with, caution should be exercised!

In this chapter, we are going to discuss some of the common alternative systems used in complimentary medicine (integrative medicine) in cancer treatment. The author does not endorse these systems or treatment options. However, there are very useful and effective herbs within these systems, and to throw out the usefulness, in my opinion, is not prudent. However, as Christian believers, it is essential to know what parts of the philosophy or practice of these cultural forms of medicine that may be potentially harmful to one's spiritual journey. So I will give you the details of these practices and then a summary of what to be careful if considering some aspects of these ancient systems of medicine. When pursuing a therapy that you are unfamiliar with, caution should be exercised. The following are the most common alternative systems of treatment.

Ayurvedic Tradition in Medical Treatment

Ayurveda is a holistic system of healing which evolved among the Brahmin sages of ancient India some 3000–5000 years ago. Ayurveda encompasses religion and philosophy as well as medicine and science. It is with the religious aspects of this system that the Christian believer should be on guard. I will define the system more specifically below. There are several aspects of this system of medicine that distinguish it from other approaches to health care:

1. It focuses on establishing and maintaining balance of the life energies within us, rather than focusing on individual symptoms.

2. It recognizes the unique constitutional differences of all individuals and therefore recommends different regimens for different types of people. Although two people may appear to have the same outward symptoms, their energetic constitutions may be very different and therefore call for very different remedies.

3. Ayurveda is a complete medical system that recognizes that ultimately all intelligence and wisdom flows from one Absolute source (Paramatman). Health manifests by the grace of the Absolute acting through the laws of Nature (Prakriti).

4. Ayurveda assists Nature by promoting harmony between the individual and Nature by living a life of balance according to her laws.

5. Ayurveda describes three fundamental universal energies that regulate all natural processes on both the macrocosmic and microcosmic levels. That is, the same energies that produce effects in the various galaxies and star systems are operating at the level of the human physiology—in your own physiology. These three universal energies are known as the Tridosha.

6. Finally, the ancient Ayurvedic physicians realized the need for preserving the alliance of the mind and body and offers

mankind tools for remembering and nurturing the subtler aspects of our humanity. Ayurveda seeks to heal the fragmentation and disorder of the mind-body complex and restore wholeness and harmony to all people.

Scope of Ayurvedic Medicine

Classically, Ayurvedic medicine was conceptualized and practiced as eight major clinical subspecialties of medicine, in addition to numerous adjunctive specialties. The eight major subspecialties continue to be taught today, and they include:

1. Internal Medicine (Kayachikitsa)

2. General Surgery (Shalya Tantra)

3. Otorhinolaryngology (Shalakya)

4. Pediatrics and Obstetric/Gynecology (Kaumarabhrtya)

5. Psychiatry (Bhutavidya)

6. Toxicology (Agada Tantra)

7. Nutrition, Detoxification, and Rejuvenation (Rasayana Tantra)

8. Fertility and Virility (Vajikarana)

For every disease, there is information about definition, etiology, prodrome, clinical symptoms, pathophysiology, prognosis, principles of treatment, medicines, diet, lifestyle recommendations, and even etymology. This approach is strikingly similar to that of modern medicine and even more comprehensive.

Over the last century, Ayurvedic medicine has experienced a rebirth and has continued to evolve its holistic approach to health in accordance with modern needs and scientific advances of the day.

The Five Elements

In Ayurveda, everything in the universe is made up of combinations of the Five Elements (Pancha Mahabhutas). This includes the human being, which also acquires a soul or spirit. These five elements are known as:

- space, or *akasha*
- air, or *vayu*
- fire, or *tejas*
- water, or *apa*
- earth, or *prithvi*

These five elements, it should be understood, derive from and are expressions of an unmanifested and undifferentiated Creative Principle, which is One. This is not the same as a Divine Creator (One True God). Ayurveda doesn't recognize an almighty creator of all that exists or a savior.

These five elements are to be understood in a material sense as well as a subtle sense. By earth, we are to understand not only the terrain of our planet or the iron in our red blood cells and spleen, but also the quality of steadfastness of mind, strength of one's moral fiber, one's slow and quiet undeterred advancement toward a goal, and the resistance to the manifestations of others.

By water, we mean to imply the cohesive aspects of reality, which flow into and hold things together, perfectly and simply witnessed in the ubiquitous H20 molecule. And the other elements too were intended by the ancient *vaidyas* (physicians) to communicate the essential universal principle inherent in a particular element.

By fire, we mean the universal force in nature that produces heat and radiates light; it is our passion to pursue, despite obstacles and delays; it is what burns away the cloak of ignorance (*avidya*) and allows the truth to shine with brilliance. Fire removes doubt from the mother-substance of the human heart and replaces it with joy.

Air is that transparent, rarefied, kinetic force that sets the universe in motion; it moves the blood through the vessels, wastes from the body, thoughts through the mind; it moves the birds to warmer climates in winter, it moves the planets around their suns. Space is the subtlest of all elements, which is everywhere and touches everything; in the mind it is the vessel that receives all impressions, in the heart space accepts love; space is receptivity and non-resistance to what is true.

Thus these Five Subtle Elements (*Pancha Mahabhutas*) form the basis for all things found in the material creation, from a grain of sand, to the complex physiology of every human being. Balancing these elements in just the right way for each unique individual is the key to maintaining health and treating disease, should it arise, whether it be physical, mental, or spiritual.

The *Tridosha*

The five elements can be seen to exist in the material universe at all scales, both organic and inorganic, from peas to planets. When they enter into the biology of a living organism, man for example, they acquire a biological form. This means that the five elements are coded into three biological forces that govern all life processes. These three forces are known as the three doshas, or simply the *tridosha*. The tridosha regulates every physiological and psychological process in the living organism. The interplay among them determines the qualities and conditions of the individual. A harmonious state of the three doshas creates balance and health; an imbalance, which might be an excess (*vrddhi*) or deficiency (*ksaya*), manifests as a sign or symptom of disease. The three doshas are known as *Vata*, *Pitta*, and *Kapha*.

You can think of these three doshas as fundamental biological energies that regulate all the life processes of an individual. And as we will discuss later, although all individuals are made up of these same three energies, we all have them in unique proportions. The doshas obtain their qualities by virtue of their elemental composition, as we can see in the simple diagram below.

Each of the three doshas is composed of two elements as shown here:

Elements composing the tridosha:

- Vata:
  space (akasha)
  air (vayu)

- Pitta:
  fire (tejas)
  water (apa)

- Kapha:
  water (apa)
  earth (prithvi)

Thus, Vata is composed of space and air, Pitta of fire and water, and Kapha of water and earth. Vata dosha has the mobility and quickness of space and air; Pitta dosha the metabolic qualities of fire and water; Kapha dosha the stability and solidity of water and earth. Interestingly, the Sanskrit entomology of the word *dosha* gives it the meaning of "blemish, that which darkens." This alerts us to the fact that when in balance these force are life supporting, but when imbalanced, they are the agents of disease and misery.

Vata dosha: The term "vata" stems from a Sanskrit word *vaayu*, which means "that which moves things"; it is sometimes translated as "wind." It is composed of the elements space and air—the lightest and subtlest of the five elements. It is considered in some ways to be the most influential of the three doshas because it is the moving force behind the other two doshas, which are incapable of movement without it. Vata dosha is responsible for all the somatic activities and sensations. It is the intelligence that channels perceptions (temperature, pressure, sweetness, lightening, violin music, etc.) through the appropriate sensory organs, converts them into internal psychological events, and then orchestrates the appropriate response via the organs of action. It is responsible for all movements in the mind and body: the movement of air in and out of the lungs, the flow of blood through the circulatory system, nutrients through the alimentary tract, and thoughts through the mind. Vata promotes a healthy balance between the thought and emotion and gives rise to creativity, activity, and clear comprehension.

Because among other functions Vata regulates the nervous processes involved with movement, thoughts, emotions, eating, drinking, elimination, and our general functioning, its disturbance can often have far-reaching consequences.

Pitta Dosha: The term "pitta" comes from the Sanskrit word *pinj*, meaning "to shine" (according to Sir Monier-Williams its exact entomology is a mystery). It carries the meaning of "that which digests" and is associated with the idea of being yellow-tinged, or bilious. In its widest sense, Paittika digestive function includes all chemical and metabolic transformations in the body as well as processes that promote heat production (i.e. conversion of iodine to triiodotyrosine in the thyroid gland). Pitta also governs our ability to digest ideas and impressions and to therefore perceive the true nature of reality. It stimulates the intellect and creates enthusiasm and determination. Pitta is often regarded as the "fire" within the body. Think of it as the energy stored in the chemical bonds of all the organic substances that makes us up; it's encoded in our hormones, enzymes, organic acids, and neurotransmitters. Charaka Samhita, an ancient Ayurvedic text, teaches that pitta functions in digestion, heat production, providing color to the blood, vision, and skin luster.

Kapha dosha: The term "kapha" derives from the Sanskrit word *shlish*, which means "that which holds things together; to embrace; coherent." In fact, one of the other designations for kapha appearing in some of the older literature is *shleshma.* It is the force that provides structure to everything from an individual atom or cell to the sturdy musculoskeletal frame. It gives strength, stability, and endurance—both physical and psychological—and promotes human emotions and capacities, such as love, compassion, empathy, understanding, forgiveness, loyalty, and patience.

One very important function of Kapha dosha in the human body is that it governs immunity and resistance against disease; its energy promotes self-healing and the ongoing processes of self-repairs of which we are largely unaware. Where Vata and Pitta effects become active in the body, Kapha acts to limit and control these two forces and prevent their excessive activity. The two *mahabhutas* that compose Kapha are water and earth. Together, these two prototypical elements form the fundamental protoplasm of life. Kapha imparts mind-body-spirit stability and resilience. It is the anabolic force in the body that governs the formation of neuropeptides, stomach linings, and all new cells and tissues of the body, which are constantly being destroyed and re-created.

Ayurvedic Concepts of Disease (the Five Elements)

The Ayurvedic definition of health is that state in which the structure and function of a particular individual is operating optimally and the individual is in a state of physical, mental, and spiritual equilibrium. Both *Charaka and Vagbhata* elegantly describe the Ayurvedic state of health:

- All three doshas are in equilibrium with regard to the individual *prakriti*

- All seven tissues, *dhatus,* are in the proper state of strength and integrity

238

- The digestive fires, *agnis,* are balanced resulting in proper appetite, digestion, and assimilation

- The waste materials, *malas,* are being produced and eliminated in a regular manner

- The sense organs, *indriyani,* are functioning normally and the mind is undisturbed

- The individual is experiencing happiness and contentment

Disease manifests as the opposite of some or all of the criteria for health listed above. It is a state of dysequilibrium of the doshas, dhatus, agnis, and malas; the individual is out of harmony both internally and with relation to the environment and experiences unpleasant sensations and misery in some form (*duhkya*).

Ayurveda asserts the truth of the principle of *svabhavo-paramavada,* which states that every living being has an inherent tendency to move in the direction of self-healing and balance. The balance toward which we naturally move is our *prakriti,* or our unique and natural proportion of Vata, Pitta, and Kapha inherited by us at birth. The disease state is known as *vikriti,* which represents a deviation from that natural proportion of the doshas. According to Ayurveda, if one lives a natural, simple, and clean life, there will always be more momentum in the direction of health than toward disease. There is an inherent tendency in Nature to move from *vikriti to prakriti,* and systems of medicine are merely strategies to assist this gentle, yet inexorable, self-healing progression.

Ayurveda recognizes the closely intertwined relationship between describing the pathological process in a person and assessing the disease state. Ayurvedic medicine demands an extensive and precise examination of the disease process and of the individual in whom it is manifesting. There are in fact no shortcuts to take to arrive at a correct diagnosis. No computerized diagnostic tools or technological imaging techniques can ever produce an accurate picture of the disease process. In order to reach an understanding of both the nature of the disease as well as the disease process in the individual, Ayurveda has evolved a unique simultaneous approach to diagnosis and pathology. This method is known as *rogi-roga pariksha.*

Ayurveda is indeed the only medical system that describes an elaborate strategy for assessing both the patient *(rogi)* and the disease *(roga)*. In contrast, allopathic (conventional medicine) medicine focuses intently on only the disease. Patients in modern hospitals are even often identified only by their particular disease as exemplified by the common query on morning rounds: "How's the gastric ulcer in Room 584 doing?" The Ayurvedic physician never regards his patient as some form of "disease entity" and always keeps in view the complete human being. This is the type of physician care all of us deserve. However, this system would be perfect if God was included as the Great Physician and Divine Healer. In every patient there is a human being; in every disease condition there is need for complete healing. The physician is the facilitator and God is the Healer.

I have outlined for you briefly a comprehensive philosophy of healing. There are many similarities in Christian healing as well. The most important point to remember is healing that is separated from God is not complete. Hopefully, you can recognize how easy it could be to be taken into a spiritual dilemma if this system can promise complete physical healing. It is true that we are all humans and not disease entities walking the planet, but it is essential to know that we are created by God. I have to emphasize that the diagnostic system of Ayurveda is thorough and more comprehensive as I mentioned above.

Summary

After reading the details, you can see how valuable a healing tradition of Ayurveda can be. However, the danger lies in the deception that it is the harmony of the body and mind alone facilitating this healing. Ayurveda as a religion leaves out the Divine Creator of heaven and Earth. The value of Ayurveda rests in the diversity of plant medicines available in East Indian tradition of medicine. The scientific system of Ayurvedic diagnosis is also extremely valuable when trying to identify the cause of disease. In my opinion, acceptance of Ayurveda as medicine and science is safe as long as the religious philosophy is not embraced. It can be very difficult in trying to determine what is spiritually safe for the Christian believer. Prayer and discernment are necessary. In addition, seeking expert advice from a physician who is knowledgeable in integrative and alternative medicine and who also is of the Christian faith would be advised. I have shared the details to enlighten and inform you so that you can make an informed and intelligent decision regarding Ayurveda and the treatment of cancer.

CHINESE TRADITION IN MEDICAL TREATMENT (TCM)

The term "traditional Chinese medicine" (TCM) is used to describe the system of medicine that has developed in China. The earliest written records of TCM date back 3,500 years, and archeological discoveries suggest the origins of TCM may stretch back at least 5,000 years.

Although it is called traditional, TCM has changed over time and is very much a part of the modern world. In its more than 2,000 years of recorded history, TCM has evolved under many influences, including politics, economics, science, technology, and social and cultural changes. At one point in its very long history, TCM came close to being officially replaced by Western medicine. With the fall of the Qing dynasty in 1911, China's leaders were intent on creating a new and modern state, and that included Western medicine. By the mid-1950s, however, traditional Chinese medicine had regained popularity, and the first four of many medical colleges were established. TCM has continued to grow as a system of medicine, and educational programs ranging from technical certificates to Ph.D's are available to students. TCM, particularly as it is practiced in China today, incorporates and adapts Western scientific and technological developments and applies them where and when appropriate.

Some Concepts in TCM

Traditional Chinese medicine is as complex and specialized as conventional medicine. Although it is impossible to summarize even the main concepts and principles in a fact sheet, we have touched briefly on some of these below.

- The idea of pairs of opposites in balance, like day and night, sun and moon, light and dark, male and female, is expressed by yin and yang. Yin and yang are sometimes graphically represented by the Taoist symbol.

- *Qi* (pronounced chee, also written *chi, or ch'i*) is often translated as vital force, or vital energy, or life force. *Qi* is both energy and matter. *Qi* flows in, around, and through the body in channels or meridians.

- The organs or organ systems of the body as described in TCM are quite different from the Western understanding. Although most organs are similar to the Western concept in name and location, in TCM they may play a different role. For example, a patient may be diagnosed by a TCM doctor as having a liver deficiency, even though the liver is perfectly normal and functional in conventional terms.

- Disease may be caused by external or internal factors. The six external causes of disease—sometimes called the six evils or six elements—are wind, cold, fire, damp, summer heat, and dryness. The internal causes of disease—sometimes translated as the seven affects—are joy, anger, anxiety, thought, sorrow, fear, and fright.

Diagnosis

A TCM doctor uses four main techniques to assess a patient and arrive at a diagnosis.

1. Visual: looking at the tongue, complexion, and skin, and observing the patient's behavior

2. Listening and smelling: listening to the quality, pitch, and tone of the patient's voice, smelling body odors

3. Questioning: asking detailed questions about the patient's symptoms, complaints, lifestyle, etc.

4. Touching: the TCM doctor is trained to assess the patient's pulse (at the wrist, through the radial artery) in a highly complex fashion, which can yield as many as twenty different pulses

Once the patient has been assessed, the TCM doctor can classify the problem and then decide on the best course of treatment. Treatment is tailored to the individual patient, depending on how the illness or complaint is classified.

Treatment and Oriental Medicine

Treatment in TCM is basically allopathic, in that conditions or diseases are treated with opposite measures. For example, a condition related to cold is treated with heat, one related to a deficit is treated with supplementation, and one related to excess is treated with drainage. The principles of treatment that guide the doctor of TCM are: treating the cause of an illness directly; treating the cause and, at the same time, supporting and encouraging the body's own ability to "cure" the illness; or supporting the body without treating the cause directly. This last approach is called *fu zheng,* which is often translated as "supporting the righteous." No matter which approach they

243

use, TCM doctors have a variety of tools and techniques for treatment. Not all TCM practitioners will use all the techniques available. Like conventional physicians, TCM doctors may specialize in certain types of diseases or treatments.

Medicine is not limited to herbs but also includes minerals and animal products. Prescriptions can be complex and may include as many as twenty or more ingredients. Some of the ingredients may treat the cause of the illness directly, others may support the body's own defenses, while still others may help reduce the side effects of other ingredients.

Medicines may be taken as teas, liquid extracts, capsules, and tablets. Although preparing teas can be time-consuming (the teas may have to be boiled, then steeped, strained, and left to cool), this may be the best way to obtain an individually tailored treatment. Some commonly used prescriptions are premixed and available as tablets. Although these are more convenient to take, the pills may not be as precise a match for a certain condition as individualized teas. Some medicines may be made from powdered ingredients that are mixed for each individual prescription and put into capsules.

Moxibustion: Moxibution refers to the burning of small amounts of dried and powdered *moxa* (a herb known as *Artemesia vulgaris, ai ye,* or mugwort) on or over the body. *Moxa* can affect the flow of qi and is often used in combination with acupuncture.

Tui Na

Although the term *Tui Na* is sometimes translated as "pushing and pulling," it really refers to a system of massage, body manipulation, and stimulation of acupuncture points by hand. Tui Na may be used to stimulate the flow of qi to treat neurological or orthopedic problems or as a substitute for acupuncture when needles may be inappropriate (for children, for example).

Qigong

Qigong (pronounced "chee goong," also written as *Chi Kung, Chi Gong, Qi Gong, etc.*) is a way of manipulating or affecting the flow of qi through exercise, breathing, and meditation. It is similar to Tai Chi, but qigong exercises are said to produce much stronger healing effects. As a daily practice, qigong may be particularly useful in maintaining good health and preventing illness.

Dietary treatment

The TCM doctor may prescribe certain foods, seasonings, or dishes that have healing properties. Other foods or alcohol may be removed from the diet to enhance healing.

Summary

After reading the details, you can see how valuable a healing tradition of Chinese medicine can be. However, the danger lies in embracing the philosophy of Buddha. This religious philosophy is work based upon practices of Chinese folklore and religion and leaves out the hope of eternal life with a loving compassionate God. It seems to appeal to the intellect, providing a sense of harmony of the body and mind to facilitate healing. Embracing Buddha as a religion leaves out the Divine Creator of heaven and Earth and the death and resurrection of His Son for the salvation of mankind.

The value of Chinese medicine rests in the diversity of plant medicines available in China and the concept of working with the sick until they are made well. The scientific system of Chinese diagnosis is also extremely valuable when trying to identify the cause of disease. In my opinion, acceptance of traditional Chinese medicine as medicine and science is safe as long as the religious philosophy is not embraced. It can be very difficult in trying to determine what is spiritually safe for the Christian believer. Prayer and discernment are necessary. In addition, seeking the expert advice from a physician who is knowledgeable in integrative and alternative medicine and who also is of the Christian faith would be advised. I have shared the details to enlighten and inform you so that you can make an informed and intelligent decision regarding traditional Chinese medicine and the treatment of cancer.

ACUPUNCTURE IN MEDICAL TREATMENT

By inserting fine needles into the body, the TCM doctor can affect the flow of qi, relieving blockages, and diverting the flow. The qi can be redirected to organs or areas of the body where there is a deficiency or away from areas where there is excess. Studies of acupuncture have shown that the treatment may stimulate the immune system by increasing the production of interferons (chemical messengers), improving the bacteria-killing ability of white blood cells and increasing the number of red blood cells. Acupuncture has also been studied as a treatment for HIV-related peripheral neuropathy. Although one large study found no significant difference in pain relief between acupuncture, standard medical treatment, and placebo, the acupuncture points studied in this trial were standardized, so that everyone received exactly the same treatment. Usually, acupuncture treatments are designed to fit the individual, and, as the researchers concluded, individualized treatments may have different effects. Unfortunately, most of the vast amount of research into TCM has been published in Chinese-language medical and scientific journals.

HOMEOPATHIC AND EUROPEAN TRADITION IN MEDICAL TREATMENT

Homeopathy is system of medicine that applies different principles than mainstream medicine. Samuel Hahnemann, a German physician of the late 1700-early 1800 era, developed homeopathy. His main purpose was to establish some validity in using substances that provoked a curative response to a number of different symptoms. He found that a tiny amount of a substance given for certain symptoms would provoke a curative action. However, when this same substance was administered to healthy individuals in higher doses it would cause the symptoms. This is where the Law of Proving came into existence. One of the first laws of homeopathy is known as the Law of Similars ("like cures like"); this is the foundational law of homeopathy and every aspect of this system builds upon it.

Practitioners of homeopathy are M.D.'s, D.O.'s, or N.D.'s that specialize in either acute conditions or more comprehensive constitutional conditions. Homeopathy should never be considered the "cure all" or "silver bullet" of all disease. Illnesses such as cancer, diabetes, chronic fatigue, serious infections, and serious injuries that require conventional medical intervention should not be treated by homeopathy alone. The aim of homeopathy is to treat the underlying cause rather than merely concentrating on a set of symptoms. Homeopathic medicines come in different potencies, depending upon the condition and practitioner's preference and success in dosage usage in the particular medical condition treated. The remedies can be made into tablet, pellets, liquid, and vaccine. High potency (i.e. more dilute) remedies are used for severe symptoms and lower potency (less dilute) for milder ones.

The homeopathic view is that during the process of healing, symptoms are redirected from more important body systems (deeper levels) to the surface systems that are less complex. The healing direction is a crucial concept in homeopathy and is known as the "Law of Cure." This simply states that healing occurs from the inside—out from the top—down and in the opposite order of how the symptoms are initially presented.

In other words, if an individual developed a skin rash and suppressed the rash by the use of something like cortisone, this action could drive the illness into a deeper level body system, such as the lung, for instance. The direct result of this action could be the development of asthma. The cortisone suppressed the rash but drove the condition deeper. When a homeopathic medicine is chosen to match the symptoms of the condition, and it is the right remedy for the condition, the rash reappears and the asthma improves. Though the rash is a troublesome symptom, it is on the surface and the body is giving a very important message that should not be suppressed. Getting the rash to go away by addressing the symptom alone is not facilitating the homeopathic Law of Cure.

In some cases there may be aggravation of symptoms by the administration of a certain homeopathic remedy. Usually, this is short-lived and will resolve. This is known as an aggravation reaction. In some cases a remedy can bring about a "healing crisis," which is the disease condition being treated worsens. This doesn't mean that the remedy is not effective; it may mean that the dosing is too strong or the frequency of the dose is too often or that the body needs a different remedy to facilitate the acceptance of the key remedy initially given.

Homeopathy requires a delicate amount of skill and should never be practiced carelessly. Experimentation in homeopathy can be harmful and present a potential obstacle to the cure. My best advice is to seek professional homeopathic expertise with ten years or greater experience in the treatment of cancer as a specialty. This system of medicine has great potential and as a whole is safe when practiced with skill and care. There are no superstitious roots in homeopathy and the fundamental laws of nature are respected. In my opinion, it is safe for the Christian to consider this as part of the overall integrative treatment plan.

NATIVE AMERICAN TRADITION IN MEDICAL TREATMENT

Native American healing is ritualistic in nature. Its origins are found in the Eurasians who crossed the land bridge of the Bering Strait that joined Siberia and Alaska. Eventually, these peoples migrated south to the Americas, particularly North America. This system of healing is based upon ancient practices and most of these practices and beliefs share characteristics that link them to the Asian healing practices.

The main features of Native American healing are the integration of medicine and religious practice, a belief of an integral relationship between the person and the environment and the universe. There is a strong belief in spiritual causes of disease and that the forces of health are governed by the spiritual health of the person. The tribal elders who may also practice Shaman rituals administer purging rituals and the use of herbs as medicine. Shamans are trained spiritual healers and often considered elders of healing.

What Is Shamanism?

Shamanism is a primitive religious system in which the shaman, or medicine man, is the central figure. It is a form of folk medicine, mind-body or trance healing, or "white magic" that relies on healer's spiritual powers. The battle is between hostile forces and the problems facing the people in the tribal community. When performing healing ceremonies, the shaman is believed to be in a trance state and is believed to be possessed by gods and spirits that act through him or her. The shaman is all-powerful at this instant and expected to restore health, protect the tribe, foretell the future, and guide and safeguard the tribal community. Shamans believe they have a special ability to communicate with the spiritual world through altered mental states. The shaman, when in this all-powerful state, becomes like a god of healing. The main objective is to promote the expectation of recovery of the patient. The spirit battle needs to be won over the evil spirits.

Modern Shaman therapy can include chanting, drumming, dancing, and spirit visualization, and is reportedly being used in clinics in the US. "Psychic surgery" is another healing force involving extraction of "tumors," in a painless and bloody "incision" in the patient's abdomen. Animal parts have been found hidden on the shamans who perform these procedures, leading to the suspicion of the credibility of the practice.

Current research evidence: There is a vast amount of historic material written over the centuries about shamanic practices. These practices have not been subject to research in establishing the efficacy of the philosophy. There aren't any current certification programs or professional associations at this time. The scientific validity of the practice is questioned and to date has no credibility. The herbal medicines utilized in Native American healing are very powerful.

Benefits and cautions for the Christian: Native American herbal tradition has contributed greatly to the use of herbs as medicines in a variety of health conditions. Discarding the philosophy and utilizing the herbs is the recommendation to the Christian believer. Christianity offers healing for body, mind, and spirit without possessive spirits and strange deities that leave an individual vulnerable to dark forces. God illuminates the spirit of man and there is healing in His presence. Nothing has to be conjured up in order for this to be experienced. It is present and available for the asking through prayer and faith. God is able to do the impossible. It is one God that heals and there are no other gods that can do this perfect work of free and wholesome healing.

The emphasis on mind control and possessive gods and spirits in the ritual of healing makes this healing philosophy very harmful to spiritual health. It is the Holy Spirit that achieves the healing work of God and not alien gods and spirits. Be cautious! New Age medicine contains elements of shamanic philosophy as well as Buddhistic practices. For the Christian it would be a potentially harmful experience!

NEW AGE MEDICINE IN MEDICAL TREATMENT

New Age medicine is a combination of different cultural religious belief systems that can include Hinduism, Buddhism, and Shamanism. The danger is that there aren't any clear boundaries, and it can be potentially harmful because of this. I have come in contact with many Christian believers that use pendulums and crystals to guide their health. The Bible takes a firm position on using methods that can conjure up alien forces that are against God's standards.

Two years ago I had a patient that phoned me in a panic and told me that she had gone to a practitioner that used therapeutic touch on her. He was not a professing Christian but was highly recommended by a Christian friend. After her therapy session, she experienced intense head pain, confusion, and anxiety. She asked me why I thought it occurred. I told her that he probably practices in a cultural belief system that is contrary to Christian belief and that the forces that command his therapy were unleashed on her. She said that this was an expensive lesson to learn because it took her several months to get better after that encounter.

There are many harmful forces in the concoction of New Age medicine. You do not need to know all of the particulars about it. Just know that it combines all of the above elements to bind and confound the soul and spirit. I have not heard of a solitary case where complete liberating healing occurred. Usually, it is a limited healing experience that keeps the soul and spirit bound to alien influences that are contrary to God.

In another case a woman came to me wanting me to solve her medical problem. In the process, she told me that she doesn't do anything that her pendulum doesn't consent to. Everything that I recommended as part of her treatment, she said her pendulum said no to. I informed this patient that I would not be able to help her if she continued to listen to her pendulum. She was upset about this. On another visit she had lost her pendulum, and this caused her to panic, because she felt this was a vital part of her healing.

This was the last time I saw this patient. God help us if we pay homage to an object rather than the Creator of all that exists! My advice to you is stay away from New Age medicine, because it blends all of the potentially dangerous spiritual techniques that can do eternal harm!

CANCER TREATMENT CLINICS IN MEXICO AND OUTSIDE THE US

A hot topic in alternative medicine is whether or not cancer treatments outside of the United States are safe and effective. Many patients I have had privilege to treat have received treatments in Mexico and South America, and many of these patients had unfavorable results. Some of the common complaints were: these clinics were not organized very well, their fees were very high ($25,000–$150,000 range), they were not sanitary, the staff could not communicate in English very well, it was difficult to communicate with once back at home, and the treatment was difficult to continue at home. In addition, some have complained of various side reactions from the therapies and were not sure exactly what the therapy was to achieve.

There are many of these clinics springing up all over in Mexico and South America because of the limitations posed in the United States, which restricts certain therapies because the FDA does not approve them. This is a very difficult situation because there are some therapies that are very promising and effective in cancer treatment but do not have sufficient amount of scientific evidence to back their efficacy. In addition, there are political reasons for restriction of these therapies, which can involve government, pharmaceutical corporations, and other interest groups. At this point, I would like to give you some effective guidelines if you are considering an out-of-the-country treatment program.

Where Is the Clinic Located?

Some of these clinics are located in Mexico, South America, and Europe. Location is an important consideration. This all depends on how ill you may be. I have had patients that have succumbed just from the trip alone. Some of the treatments in these foreign countries are not permitted in the US. They may be very difficult to continue because the products may not be permitted across the borders. Some of these foreign clinics are not easily accessible, and this is a definite point that needs further research before making any advances and decisions to enroll in the treatment program.

Who Are the Physicians and Professional Staff Members?

My advice is that the physicians that are participating in your healing must be well qualified and trained. They should be professional physicians that specialize in integrative medicine. This means blending both the best of conventional medicine and natural medicine. Quackery is prevalent in these parts and caution and care must be taken in order to keep safe. Check out the professionals and the staff. Ask for patient testimonials, and be sure that any recommendations are made from those you trust and respect.

Do They Communicate in English?

A common complaint I have received is that the doctors were excellent and the supportive staff lacking. Much of this has to do with the communication and quality standards within the organization. The clinics should have staff that communicates in English and should provide professional information including brochures, a web page, and a DVD of facilities and mode of operation so you can get a picture of what to expect. Even with this in hand, I would not make a decision based on the material you receive. A personal visit should be made by either you or a loved one to get an accurate picture of what is happening. I can tell you that many of the clinics are not following good quality standards. There are a few that I am aware of that do. The Internet is a good way to begin the search.

What Type of Therapies Are Offered?

There are many therapies and some make claims that are not legitimate. It is essential to know the type of treatment modalities that are offered. Ask for sample treatment plans that have been used with good outcomes on patients treated. Safety and efficacy are the most important factors in receiving treatment.

Are They Clean?

Many clinics outside of the US are not regulated by strict guidelines. It then becomes necessary for you to assure your own health and safety. There aren't any good rating systems in place currently, and this is an aspect that should be a priority. It is all by word of mouth and experience. The treatment facility must be clean and orderly. This reflects the type of quality care that will be received.

What Is the Cost of Treatment?

As mentioned earlier, the cost of treatment can be quite costly. You may be able to receive the same type of treatment closer to home and for a fraction of the cost.

How Effective Is the Treatment?

Talk with people who received treatment from the center of choice. This will give information that will assist you in making an informed decision. Claims are made, but you need to see proof. The most important factor is that you are at peace with the information you receive, there is a proof of efficacy, and you are comfortable with the surroundings.

Any Incidence of Harm Reported or Documented?

A good way to evaluate safety, quality, and efficacy is to take note of any harmful events reported. This is a very important factor in reaching your final decision. A good rule to follow is that if any harmful events were reported ask how many, what they were, and the end result. If the end result was the patient died, that is not good. A little bit of common sense keeps danger away.

What Is the Follow Up Treatment, and Can I Continue at Home?

Follow up treatment is very important. I have had patients receive treatment in clinics outside of the US and they could not continue the treatment for one reason or another. Be sure that the treatment can follow you and that your physician at home can appropriately administer care. A good rule here is that your physician develops a partnership as a team player to assure that you have continuity of care.

Finally, it is important to know that the treatment and program is the right choice for the type of cancer and person. For instance, the Gerson Program would be very difficult for an individual that is not compliant. This can become the obstacle to healing. There must be compatibility between the person and the method of treatment to some extent. Don't feel pressured into anything. Evaluate all of your information and options available and make it a concentrated prayer effort. When you seek divine guidance, the best options become available to you!

EVALUATING THERAPIES FROM A CHRISTIAN PERSPECTIVE

Determine the guiding principles of the therapy selected. One of the most important to consider when choosing an alternative therapy is will it harm you spiritually. An individual can be promised that a certain therapy will provide physical healing, but if this is at the detriment or harm of the spirit, then this will become a damaging experience. It is difficult and can be confusing when choosing an alternative therapy. Not all of these therapies are spiritually harmful and many of them offer sound principles. It is essential to search out the therapy. Pray specifically that God would reveal to you the potential dangers, and if your spirit is uneasy after you have gathered the facts, regardless of who has been healed or helped, don't do it! Good rules to follow are:

1. Are the claims legitimate and realistic?

2. Does it fit in with being a good steward of health and well-being?

3. Is it consistent with the principles found in God's Word?

4. Does it violate the principles of God?

5. Does it violate my sense of peace?

6. Does it cause confusion and agitation within?

If any of the above questions are answered yes, then consider potential harm as a possible outcome. Prayer and careful counsel are necessary in making a peaceful decision. My suggestion is that you ask God to lead you to a physician that specializes in integrative care that also has a strong faith in God and is a true servant of the Lord. They are out there and God can pave the way. It has been my goal and purpose to establish God-centered integrative health care clinics throughout the US. Pray for me as I work to fulfill God's mission!

Chapter 14

The Journey Toward Healing

The body is one unit, though it is made up of many cells, and though all its cells are many, they form one body. . . . If the white cell should say, because I am not a brain cell, I do not belong in the body, it would not for that reason cease to be part of the body. And if the muscle cell should say to the optic nerve, because I am not an optic nerve, I do not belong to the body, it would not for that reason cease to be part of the body. If the whole body were an optic nerve cell, where would be the ability to walk? If the whole body were an auditory nerve, where would be the sense of sight? But in fact God has arranged the cells in the body, every one of them, just as he wanted them to be. If all cells were the same, where would the body be? As it is, there are many cells, but one body

—Dr. Paul Brand

The road is hard, the journey swift as we travel toward the grave. This body will return to dust, But what of the soul to save?

—Selected

Where Healing Begins

Then shall thy light break forth as the morning and thine health shall spring forth speedily and thy righteousness shall go before thee; the glory of the Lord shall be thy reward. . . . And the Lord shall guide thee continually, and shall satisfy thy soul in drought, and make fat thy bones; and thou shall be like a watered garden, and like a spring of water, whose waters fail not. And they that shall be of thee shall build the old waste places; thou shat raise up the foundations of many generations; and thou shall be called, The repairer of the breach, The restorer of paths to dwell in. (Isaiah 58: 8, 11–12)

Understand the Concept

Understanding the concept of healing is the starting point of the journey toward healing. Healing is a process that is orchestrated by God and experienced by mankind. Healing can occur over time or as a miraculous instantaneous work. The miracle healing is just as prevalent today as it was for the apostolic age.

There are many avenues that an individual can take to experience true healing. Often it is not any one isolated event that we can put our finger on that offers such healing. However, there is one single truth that all can affirm and that is that healing begins on a personal level. I have observed in many individuals this single truth and have seen different dimensions of healing through their journeys. Individuals that are experiencing suffering in their physical, emotional, and spiritual health will often gravitate to resources that offer some explanation for the purposes of suffering. Such suffering often allows for deep reflections of what it means to live in the moment.

Creativity and a compassionate love will replace depression and self-pity when the focus is turned to others. There are some very essential points to ponder that move an individual toward liberation of soul and spirit even when encountering physical suffering. It is often physical suffering that prompts deeper attention to the central core of life, which is housed in the soul and spirit.

We Are in the Age of Miracles

One of the main defenses against false healing is the true miracle of healing. There are many systems of healing today that offer the false assurance of completeness away from God. These systems emphasize body and mind interaction, and they usually don't clearly define the importance of the unity of body, soul, and spirit in light of total dependence upon divine sustenance. This is the result of an incomplete understanding of the spirit, soul, and body interaction from God's perspective. God's foundational perspective of healing is demonstrated with intensity and power because of His presence. The great pioneers of faith found in the Bible and through the history of the Christian Church demonstrated and perpetuated the gift of healing. This miracle is intensely alive today but craftily hidden by adversarial counterfeits. Unfortunately, it is the human element that often obstructs the healing forces of God. The focus shifts to what gives immediate relief.

Moreover, what we see even more so today is the shift from a dependence upon some medication to fix the problems that afflict the spirit or soul to a therapy or meditative force that yields a façade of psycho emotional euphoria. This results from the realization that there are no miracle medicines that one can physically take to remedy the pain encountered in the soul and spirit parts. To give attention to these pains may spark some sort of conviction that one refuses to face. In other words, this reflects the need to heal from the *inside out*. Most systems in practice today focus in upon the *outside in*. The Bible tells us that those things that trouble us are housed on the *inside*. The "outside in" concept of healing offers a plethora of coping strategies that focus in upon the externals of an individual, which in some way effect how the interaction between self, others, and the world environment is to occur.

A changing environment requires a better method of coping with the pain—a pragmatic method (an evolutionary process) that is cause and effect experimentation and is based upon individual philosophical belief rather than on principle.

Inside Out	**Outside In**
(God-centered vertical healing)	(Man-centered horizontal healing)
• Unchangeable principles of God	• Focus on cause and effect
• Origin is from Omnipotent Creator	• Evolutionary philosophically based system
• Is a free gift to all who accept	• Seeks global and cultural acceptance
• Based upon truth (consistent)	• Pragmatic (whatever works is true)

Our Healing Is Our Need

In our need for the healing touch of the Master, we must acknowledge and act by faith and trust that this need will be met. With God there aren't any cases of failure. With faith there are no failures. Healing is not always instantaneous, and sickness or suffering lie with a specific purpose of God that needs to be made manifest or with incomplete faith, trust, and/or defective knowledge. Sickness doesn't always have a negative connotation but may be for the demonstration of the grace and divine comfort and care.

We Need to See a Living Christ

Every generation needs a living Christ and every community needs the signs of healing to confirm the promises found in the Word. Hebrews 2:4: "God bears witness, both with signs and wonders . . . . And gifts of the Holy Ghost, according to His own will." Jesus did not say, "*I will* be with you alway." He said: "*I am.*"—Matthew 28:20 (Italics mine) His standard does not change. So it is not simply "healing" but *power* to be well, and it is as free now as ever.

The Great Physician Heals

Jesus healed the multitude; we read this in Matthew 8:16. Jesus healed all those who had need and did it on the Sabbath to boot. Through this He proved that healing was not of a secular nature or apart from the administrative work of God. Healing is a holy and sacred work that is remains unified with God's higher purpose for man. This healing offered salvation of the soul and restoration, not for professional treatment or reimbursement. The Bible mentions few doctors and the coverage is usually one of discouraging results. As a matter of fact, Luke left medicine to become an evangelist and to accompany the apostle Paul in his travels. It was comforting to know that a physician was present. However, he observed more miracles thorough the power of the Holy Spirit than he had opportunity to administer with medicine. This doesn't mean that there is no use for physicians. It simply means that there is need for a new type of physician, one who allows the supernatural force of God to work the miracle and to be the vehicle that can facilitate this healing power. This will involve the expenditure of soul and spiritual energy and greater faith, trust, prayer, and commitment to God.

Healing Requires Empathetic Interaction

Usually, the individual who is overcome with illness becomes aware of the deeper significance and purpose of life. The healer needs to be able to understand the needs of individuals that need healing and relate to the pain and be willing to offer solutions that often require soul and spirit expenditure, similar to the way Jesus did when He healed the woman with the issue of blood.

Charles Spurgeon gives an empathetic account of what it is like to administer the gift of healing: (Charles Spurgeon Sermons)

That it might be fulfilled which was spoken by Esaias the prophet, saying, Himself took our infirmities, and bare our sicknesses. (Matthew 8:17)

First, he bare our sicknesses by intense sympathy. When Christ looked at all those sick people, he did, as it were, take all their sicknesses upon himself. You know what I mean. If you talk with a person who is very ill, and you feel for him, you seem to lay his pains upon yourself, and then you have power to comfort him. When I am seeing troubled people, I enter into one sorrowful case after another till I am more sad than any of them. I try as far as I can to have fellowship with the case of each one, in order to be able to speak a word of comfort to him; and I can say, from personal experience, that I know of nothing that wears the soul down so fast as the outflow of sincere sympathy with the sorrowing, desponding, depressed ones. I have sometimes been the means in God's hand of helping a man who suffered with a desponding spirit; but the help I have rendered has cost me dearly. Hours after, I have been myself depressed, and I have felt an inability to shake it off. You and I have not a thousandth part of the sympathy that was in Christ. He sympathized with all the aggregate of human woe, and so sympathized that he made his heart a great reservoir into which all streams of grief poured themselves. My Master is just the same now. Though he is in heaven, he is just as tender as he was on earth. Healing is a journey involving our spirit and soul; without their involvement, the body cannot heal.

Trust or Worry?

Ask, and it shall be given you; seek and ye shall find; knock and it shall be opened unto you. (Luke 11:9)

The only limiting factor in not being able to receive any good and constructive blessing in life, particularly in keeping good health, is the human factor. We have all heard the saying, "To err is human," and all humans on the face of the planet at some time or another have fallen into the category of "to err."

Francis of Assisi many centuries ago recognized that there was a natural tendency within him to be overly concerned about his selfish ambition in life. This troubled him on many occasions and it continued until he did something about it. On one occasion, he had his heart fixed on defending his province in order to be top dog and in favor with Roman Church authorities. This he felt was a good pursuit because everything within him stood firm to defend God and country. What better achievement could there possibly be?

Francis, though busy with his earthly endeavors, was then contacted by the highest authority known in all of creation. The simple words from God came to Francis: "Why give service to the servant when you can serve the Master alone?" (The Life of Saint Francis; Brother Thomas of Celano, Assisi, Italy) Of course, immediately, through divine guidance, Francis knew that Jesus was calling him to service, and he left his fishing net behind and became a fisher of men. Similar stories can be found in the history of the Christian Church. What did Francis learn? He learned to become totally dependent upon his Creator for everything. His anxiety about life was converted into an assurance that cannot be known apart from God. This is reflected in his simple prayer:

> Lord, make me an instrument of your peace. Where there is hatred let me sow love. Where there is injury pardon. Where there is discord unity. Where there is doubt faith. Where there is error truth. Where there is despair hope. Where there is sadness joy. Where there is darkness light. O Divine Master, grant that I may not so much seek to be consoled as to console. To be understood as to understand. To be loved as to love. For it is in giving that we receive. It is in pardoning that we are pardoned. It is in dying that we are born to eternal life.
>
> —Francis of Assisi

What can I do with my worry? *Worry* is a paralyzing word that is experienced by countless numbers of people everyday. Worry negatively affects health. Worry is linked to panic disorders and uncontrollable emotions. Worry can cause illnesses like cancer and can contribute to high blood pressure and heart disease. It can also cause cases of extreme fatigue and loss of health. There is never an end to the things one can worry about. Some of the more common things to worry about include death, loss, health, finances, relationships, and the future.

I would like to guide you along in understanding the origins of worry. The following comparisons have helped me in many ways and continue to assist me in converting worry into manageable concerns of life. It is essential to understand the origins, destinations, and foundational aspects of life experience, and the following may assist you in understanding this concept. Let's create a comparison chart.

Heaven Bound	Earth Bound
• Vertical thinking (God-centered)	• Horizontal thinking (human-centered) Unbelief
• Faith	• Worry
• Trust	• Self-ambition (no room for others)
• Priorities (think of others)	• Inaction (senseless situation ethics)
• Action (purpose in life)	

Ephesians 4:10 illustrates the larger purpose of life: "He that descended is the same also that ascended up far above all the heavens that he might fill all things." When our focus is on things that are earthbound, we are living life in a descent pattern. We are bound by horizontal thinking that can only see things from the perspective of man rather than God. Vertical thinking looks to the Divine Creator and yields eternal value that cannot be measured in earthly terms. The Earth scenario is one of confinement, walls of defense, and localities (living

from situation to situation) that can lock us in a box. This is where an individual can be subject to thinking within the box.

There seems to be some kind of false security that comes along with this. I would call it fear. What kind of fear? The fear of losing the approval of authorities, friends, co-workers, thereby, losing self-worth. Fear and worry are partners when it comes to crippling trust and faith. There is a risk in coming out of this horizontal box-like thinking and becoming a vertical out-of-box individual. You may have to develop new friendships, change employment, and take new action in how you communicate, but you will attain a new freedom. These changes in communication will be based upon a new sense of confidence rather than a place of inferiority.

- Vertical thinking—Think of it a new model of communication based upon vertical thinking. This is seeing God's higher purpose in your life. He has already given you the resources. He is waiting for you to ask and implement.

- Faith—Faith is the realization that God will and has performed all that He has promised. This will continue to become evident throughout human existence. This new communication is based upon knowing that all that is contained within your life-experience will work out for the good of all involved.

- Trust—probably the biggest challenge is the stabilizing element. I will elaborate on this later.

- Priorities—having a sense of service. This is not self-centered focus but rather a broader vision that includes benevolence and humanitarian action. Self-ambition focuses upon what I can get out of it rather than what I can contribute. This in the long run yields a lasting work of posterity. It is not a labor of recognition alone. It is a continuous self-less focus. It may seem at times that your labor is obscure. However, there is a light that rises from obscurity. Abraham Lincoln is a prime example of this. He was born in an obscure place and suffered many defeats before becoming the greatest President of the United States. This is a common story of most men and women of greatness. If you were to ask them about the main ingredient that contributed to their greatness, they probably would tell you the ability to overcome obstacles, take action on matters that are within their control, and develop strong trust in God.

- Action—Bring your vulnerabilities to the One who has the power to do something about them. Being that He can do something about them, He will in turn give you the insight and confidence to do something about the things that touch your life.

Some helpful hints in overcoming worry.

1. Develop a worry list—Identify the things you worry about and generate a list outlining specifics about each. When you see it plainly in front of you, recognition of the depth of the worry begins to materialize. Here is a sample worry list.

   Things I am worried about:
   - health of a loved one
   - my job or business
   - finances
   - soured friendships
   - future goals
   - family relationships
   - church relationships

2. Develop a prayer list—Convert your worry list into active prayer, making your request known to God who can do something about them. Here is a sample prayer list based upon the above worries.

- Provide healing of body, soul, and spirit of this loved one and help me to be a source of encouragement, service, and love.

- Help me to be a stabilizing influence in the job or business that I am currently in. Lead me into Your purpose and ministry for my life, and help me above all to model the character of Jesus in my current experience and in future opportunities.

- I realize that Your resources are abundant. Teach me responsible ways to manage the resources You have entrusted to me. Help me to be the good steward You desire throughout this life journey.

- My heart aches because of friends I have lost for whatever reason. Help me to be open to the areas I need to change to mend friendships, and I forgive those who have wronged me and maintain false perceptions.

- Guide me in future opportunities. Help me to leave the future events with you. These are beyond my control. Help me to rely on the grace and prudence that You provide each day. Help me to be the salt of the earth and the light of the world today—tomorrow has enough troubles.

- I ask You, O Lord, to intervene on delicate family matters. I ask You to rescue and bring each in my family who do not know You in a personal way to a personal commitment to You. Speak to them in a way that they can understand through the guidance of the Holy Spirit. May Jesus become their personal Guide and Friend.

- I ask You, O Lord, to intervene in complicated matters within the church. The church is Your ultimate concern, and I acknowledge that Your grace and guidance is sufficient. Help me to take action in matters that you give me liberty in and to leave with You particulars that only You can change. Help me to rise above the conflict and obstacles to achieve Your purpose, regardless.

3. Develop an action list—Developing an action list takes paralyzing anxiety and coverts it to a manageable concern for the responsibilities of life. Here is a sample action list.

- Health needs—Identify the needs and provide for those needs appropriately with sensitivity and balance.

- Develop effective communication strategies and become a person of influence. Any classes or programs to help you should be considered and move forward in developing an effective leadership model by becoming a person of influence.

- Develop strategies to get out of debt and make prudent investment choices. Be mindful of what it means to be a steward of the blessings God has provided and move on.

- Become a better friend to those you have wronged; ask forgiveness and move on. If you have outgrown old friends, then make new friends. Forgive those old friends for their misperceptions and move on.

- Be open to God's direction for your future. Discover where your aptitude is. God is interested in helping you to achieve your heart's desire. Through prayer and action, God will assist you in discovering where you would be most fulfilled, content, and proficient. Outline a plan of action and move on.

- Identify the area you can become the greatest influence in family and church matters. Take action under God's guidance in areas that need action through prayerful direction. Don't be a box thinker. If you are a box thinker, get out of the box. Take the risk and develop your ministry under God's leadership. If the box thinkers want to remain stuck, then move on.

Transforming worry into complete trust.

Trust in the Lord with all of thine heart, and lean not unto thine own understanding. In all thy ways acknowledge him, and he shall direct thy paths. (Proverbs 3:5) Let's create another comparison chart.

Heaven	Earth
• Freedom in Spirit and Soul	• Confinement
• (Outside the box)	• (In the box)
• Total Fulfillment	• Walls of Defense
• (Ascending)	• (Descending)
• Unlimited Possibilities	• Localities
• (Complete faith)	• (Victim of circumstance)

Trust is a quality that should grow throughout life. However, it is what we trust in that can pave the way to either greater blessing or potential disaster. The best way to achieve a goal is to develop trust. The most effective way to move through the obstacles of life is by trust. Trust operates in the present tense. It possesses and receives what is promised and moves forward to conquer the mountains of life. In order for trust to develop, there has to be faith, the kind of faith in God's ability to work all things out for the good and benefit of the whole of all that touches your life. This is a very difficult concept to grasp.

In Luke 18:18–30, Jesus talked about this same challenge with a young man who was very wealthy and didn't have any need for any to help him. This man had everything that one could want in the day in which he lived. However, he comes to Jesus and asks, "What must I do to have this eternal treasure You speak of?" He wanted this treasure. He had every other kind of treasure, and it seemed as though this type of treasure was not attainable by the same means he was accustomed to. Jesus told him that he was to follow the commandments, and the young man assured Him that he did these things from his youth. Then Jesus replied to this young man and said that he lacked one thing. He said, "Sell all that you have and distribute it to the poor, and you shall have treasure in heaven, and come and follow Me."

The young man went away defeated because he had such great trust in his wealth that he wasn't ready to sacrifice it all for Jesus. Jesus was basically telling him that he was to cease putting all of his reliance upon earthly things that can only inherit the wind. Jesus was telling him of a sure trust that doesn't fade when his earthly existence comes to a close. In the same passage, Jesus assured those who heard the young man's instruction and affirmed that the things that are impossible with men are possible with God. He further stated that there is not one individual who if he were to leave all behind for the kingdom of God's sake that would be left lacking. Jesus was saying that if your trust is in the things of God, you shall receive many more blessings at this present time than you have, and what's more, you shall receive the blessings of all eternity.

What an incredible promise! Can you see the larger purpose of God? Trust sees God doing things here and now. God's way is invisible to man unless man is ready to receive such a great blessing. Trust realizes that God has done things and regards them as being already done. It's not just a bunch of promises that never come to fulfillment. Let's talk about how this new type of trust can liberate you and transform the old patterns into new freedom.

When we develop trust in God, we are able to begin to discern those on Earth worthy of our trust. We experience a freedom in the soul and spirit that removes insecurities and confinement. We no longer will settle for being inside the box. We ascend and have fulfillment in life. We no longer view obstacles as defeat, but rather we keep our eyes on the goal. Henry Ford once said "Obstacles are the frightful things that happen when we take our eyes off of the goal." What can we expect from developing such a dynamic trust? Unlimited possibilities are the result of complete trust. Trust operates in the present tense and embraces things promised. Faith can move mountains only when there is complete, unwavering trust. Total crisis is the result when trust diminishes, which leads to weakness of faith and a lack of prayerfulness in life. The walls of defensiveness are broken, and circumstantial living becomes a thing of the past.

Talk to the One who cares about your cares. "Be anxious for nothing, but in everything by prayer and supplication, with thanksgiving, let your requests be made known unto to God; and the peace of God which surpasses all understanding, will guard your hearts and minds through Christ Jesus" (Philippians 4:6–7). Bring it all to the One who can give you the solution, the keys, the resolution, and the peace! Follow as I pray with you for God's complete peace over all of the anxieties that you face just now.

A HELPFUL PRAYER

O God, I lift to You the greatest concerns of life. Take the anxieties of life and convert them into trust and peace. Through it all, help me to be mindful of the things I need to change in order to be a better servant of You. Help me to get out of the box and to be open in faith to whatever improvements You desire for me. Help me to look up and to ascend to Your throne through faith, prayer, and complete trust, with every obstacle and challenge of life I may experience. As the Serenity Prayer says: "God grant me the serenity to accept things I cannot change, the courage to change the things I can, and the wisdom to know the difference." Transform my worry into trust and peace that I may glorify You in all things. In Jesus' trusted and blessed name I pray, Amen!

THE ROAD TO HEALING

When we experience pain, most of us want immediate relief. However, there are deeper pains that lodge within us and fester over time, causing more devastating illness, including the loss of hope and spiritual death. Total healing is not just relief from physical suffering. Even when we continue to suffer from physical ailments, we can experience healing on a soul and spiritual level. Medical science tells us there are many incurable diseases, including cancer. Most of these diseases kill the body. However, medical science does not deal with the diseases of the spirit and soul—the very essence of life. Where are we to turn when we are given crushing news about our health? The natural human tendency is to react rather than respond. When diagnosed with cancer, we often react with fear instead of responding in faith.

Cancer is an illness that can steal the essence of life and breed a hopelessness that takes away the life of the soul and spirit. I have many patients who are fighting cancer. I have very few patients who give up. The key word is to *fight*. Life is worth the battle against a potentially fatal illness. But how do we fight? To whom do we turn when our defenses are weak? We must turn to the supernatural existence of God. We must reach out to God and ask for His divine intervention through prayer and diligent search. We must search for the answers He gives through His Word (the Holy Bible) and the guidance He gives through others whom we trust, whether it is family, a friend, a physician, or a clergyman. God gives life and He gives it abundantly! When we take the steps allowing God to bring healing to our innermost being, we can have the assurance that the final outcome is an excellent one.

WHICH PATH TO FOLLOW?

Believe that life is worth living and your belief will help create the fact.

—William James

To be healed from sickness and disease, we must focus on the precious gift of life. We must turn away from our old patterns of living and be transformed into a new existence. This transformation will include life-giving fruits, such as love, peace, joy, kindness, and faith. We must have faith! Jesus taught: *"For verily I say unto you, That whosoever shall say unto this mountain, Be thou removed, and be thou cast into the sea; and shall not doubt in his heart, but shall believe that those things which he saith shall come to pass; he shall have whatsoever he saith"* Italics mine (Mark 11:23).

Faith is believing that we will possess what we hope for. Faith healing is not superstition nor is it accomplished through the efforts of a single person. Healing comes from God and God alone. There is a woman mentioned in the Bible who had a bleeding disorder for many years. She had gone to many physicians and was helped by none of them. She said, "If I may touch but his clothes, I shall be whole" (Mark 5:25–28). She persisted until she saw herself well. What a powerful example of faith. The key is to believe in the source of all-perfect healing—God Himself!

There are many healers in our day and age. Many of them draw from powers that are dark and oppressive. I call these types pseudo-healers (false healers). My friends, this type of healing is temporary and may last for a moment of time. However, the healing that comes from God is for all eternity and there are no negative effects associated with it. Latch on to the power of God and cry out to Him for your complete healing. Trust Him, for He is able to do more than we could ever expect.

THE BEST SOURCE OF MEDICINE

Looking to medical science alone for answers to our deepest needs is a waste of precious life energy. The very best source of medicine comes from God's Word. In Proverbs 4:20–22, the Scripture tells us that the words spoken from the mouth of God are life giving.

Reading and growing in God's Word is the best medicine any of us can get. This doesn't mean that we discard the best that medicine has to offer. The Word of God will help us to know what is the best course for our healing. What action would be appropriate and have the best outcome? How do I proceed? When we are diligent students of His Word, we learn wisdom and we gain understanding. The Holy Spirit gives us guidance and keeps us from potential harm. Not only is our faith in His healing ability made stronger, but also our understanding deepens and we develop prudence in our decision making. The Word of God is the first source of medicine.

ANGER AND FORGIVENESS

Yesterdays are a thing of the past. Most of the time anger is generated over past failures or hurts. I was just viewing a biography on the life of President Richard Nixon. He had many set backs in his political life. He would not let the yesterdays rest. During public appearances, he would affirm that it was essential not to be defeated by issues of the past. However, during his times alone, he became very melancholy over what the press had done to him, what his political rivals did to him, and what the people of America did to him. He didn't let it go and became embittered, enraged, and depressed. This is what shattered his life, health, and happiness. The power of forgiveness is stronger and provides a way out of this. The power of forgiveness offers healing and the ability and power to forgive. To be forgiven and to forgive are the two most life giving gifts given to us by the Master Forgiver!

Oswald Chambers, an influential devoted follower of God, illustrates for us the power of God's forgiveness through the work of His Son Jesus Christ. God's interest is to restore a life and renew it. When battling cancer, life must be restored, peace offered, and anger over the past resolved. What incredible words of inspiration!

> And I will restore to you the years that the locust hath eaten, the cankerworm, and the caterpillar, and the palmerworm, my great army which I sent among you. (Joel 2:25)

> Through the Redemption God undertakes to deal with a man's past, and He does it in two ways: by forgiving him, and by making the past a wonderful culture for the future. The forgiveness of God is a bigger miracle than we are apt to think. It is impossible for a human being to forgive; and it is because this is not realised that we fail to understand that the forgiveness of God is a miracle of Divine grace. Do I really believe that God cannot, dare not, must not forgive me my sin without its being atoned for? If God were to forgive me my sin without its being atoned for, I should have a greater sense of justice than God. It is not that God says in effect, "I will pay no more attention to what you have done." When God forgives a man, He not only alters him but transmutes what he has already done. Forgiveness does not mean merely that I am saved from sin and made right for heaven; forgiveness means that I am forgiven into a recreated relationship to God.

Do I believe that God can deal with my "yesterday," and make it as though it had never been? I either do not believe He can, or I do not want Him to. Forgiveness, which is so easy for us to accept, cost God the agony of Calvary. When Jesus Christ says, "Sin no more," He conveys the power that enables a man not to sin any more, and that power comes by right of what He did on the Cross.

That is the unspeakable wonder of the forgiveness of God. To-day men do not bank on what Jesus Christ can do, or on the miraculous power of God; they only look at things from their side—"I should like to be a man or a woman after God's heart, but look at the mountain of my past that is in the way." God has promised to do the thing which, looked at from the basis of our own reason, cannot be done. If a man will commit his "yesterday" to God, make it irrevocable, and bank in confidence on what Jesus Christ has done, he will know what is meant by spiritual mirth—"Then was our mouth filled with laughter, and our tongue with singing." Very few of us get there because we do not believe Jesus Christ means what He says. "It is impossible! Can Jesus Christ re-make me, with my meanness and my criminality; re-make not only my actual life, but my mind and my dreams?" Jesus said, "With God all things are possible." The reason God cannot do it for us is because of our unbelief; it is not that God won't do it if we do not believe, but that our commitment to Him is part of the essential relationship.— Oswald Chambers (The Complete Works of Oswald Chambers; Discovery House Publishers).

Don't hang on to the pain of the past any longer. Let it go! Let it go! And let God move you and heal you of the deepest wounds. Let Him make you whole!

PRAYER: THE BEST STRATEGY

Our healing is not only a journey, but also a battle. In the Book of Job, we have a clear illustration of the battle that is waged for our very existence. This battle for life must be fought with powerful methods. Prayer is the most essential method we have. God is our only true source of life, and He alone has the power over it. God is aware of the battle; and through prayer, we liberate His power to defeat the unseen forces of evil. He does battle for us! He did battle for Job! Read the Book of Job. It is an intriguing account of God's power, deliverance, and healing. This battle is won by the strongest methodology there is—prayer!

E. M. Bounds a prayer warrior of the nineteenth and earlier twentieth century states: "Everything was possible to the men and women who knew how to pray, and it is still possible today. Prayer, indeed opened a limitless storehouse, and God's hand withheld nothing. Prayer introduced those who practiced it into a world of privilege, and brought the strength and wealth of heaven down to the aid of finite man. What rich and wonderful prayer they had who had learned the secret of victorious approach to God!"

It is essential in prayer to remember that through the power of God the battle is won. In and of ourselves, we are powerless. We must do all we can, but the power to overcome belongs to God; and when we rely upon Him, we find deliverance from the oppressive forces of sickness and disease. Our prayers do not have to be complicated dissertations, but rather, simple words of faith.

A Prayer of Healing

Oh God, provide Your complete healing and deliverance from this affliction and restore me physically, emotionally, and spiritually. Facilitate Your healing energy within my body, and renew every cell and body system, through the name and power of Jesus Christ and the power of His blood.

Holy Spirit, I cry out to you in time of this affliction. I know that I am within Your care, and that this affliction will eventually reveal a greater purpose of God in my life journey. Manifest Your comforting presence and give me faith, grace, and strength to stand, and may all who see me see You. Protect me from false perceptions and judgments of others. Remove from me the constant desire to vindicate myself, and may your divine truth be manifested. For this present suffering doesn't compare with what the Lord Jesus Christ has accomplished for me on the cross! Into Your hands I commit this fragile life and wait for Your healing. Replace this broken down body with Your wholeness and renewed strength. You love and accept me as I am. All of my imperfections and weaknesses are before You. Yet You unconditionally love me and adopt me as Your own. For You say in Your

Word that Your strength is made perfect in weakness. Thank you, God, for loving me as I am and giving me more of Your grace to overcome. I claim Your Word and pray these things in the power of the Holy Spirit, Amen!

THE HEALING LOVE OF GOD

The wonderful love of God that accepts us where we are and gives us the best of His nature. When you are lonely and forsaken, the perfect gentleman fatherhood of God and the loving mother's heart of God comforts, cares, rescues, and stabilizes. God meets us where we are. Jesus stands at the door and knocks the Bible tells us. There is no intrusion or invasion of privacy. The boundaries are not violated. He gently and lovingly comes and asks to be invited in to fill that lonely arid place. He transforms and restores with the streams of gentle love and holds our hand, walks along with us, and even carries us when we are weak. What other friend will do this all for you? When others fail you He sustains. When others disappoint He encourages. When others hurt He heals. When the burden becomes too great He carries. Embrace the love of God and take it into the loneliest place of your heart. You will find the Friend of all friends and the greatest love of all! Jesus the Risen Lord gives the greatest love that heals a multitude of hurts!

THE HEALING REST OF GOD

Come unto me, all *ye* that are weary and heavy laden, and I will give you rest. (Matthew 11:28)

God has outlined for us an absolute concept of rest. It is for the weary, burdened, and distressed. I say that this is an absolute concept because the principles of it do not change. The catch is that this rest cannot be purchased with money. It is not a vacation to the Bahamas. It is not sleeping fourteen hours a day. Another human does not extend it. God's blessing of rest is extended through divine resources. A perfect illustration of this is found in the prophet Elijah's life experience. Elijah was tired and worn out from the heavy burdens that he carried for many years. He was human and there was no possible way that this shouldering of the heavy burdens could continue. The most comforting aspect of this man's journey is that God knew he needed this perfect rest! This did not escape God's watchful eye. The following passage 1 Kings 17:1–16 outlines this for us:

> And Elijah the Tishbite, who was of the inhabitants of Gilead, said unto Ahab, As the Lord God of Israel liveth, before whom I stand, there shall not be dew nor rain these years, but according to my word. And the word of the Lord came unto him, saying, Get thee hence, and turn thee eastward, and hide thyself by the brook Cherith, that is before Jordan. And it shall be, that thou shalt drink of the brook; and I have commanded the ravens to feed thee there. So he went and did according unto the word of the Lord: for he went and dwelt by the brook Cherith, that is before Jordan. And the ravens brought him bread and flesh in the morning, and bread and flesh in the evening; and he drank of the brook. And it came to pass after a while, that the brook dried up, because there had been no rain in the land. And the word of the Lord came unto him, saying, Arise, get thee to Zarephath, which belongeth to Zidon, and dwell there: behold, I have commanded a widow woman there to sustain thee. So he arose and went to Zarephath. And when he came to the gate of the city, behold, the widow woman was there gathering of sticks: and he called to her, and said, Fetch me, I pray thee, a little water in a vessel, that I may drink. And as she was going to fetch it, he called to her, and said, Bring me, I pray thee, a morsel of bread in thine hand. And she said, As the Lord thy God liveth, I have not a cake, but an handful of meal in a barrel, and a little oil in a cruse: and, behold, I am gathering two sticks, that I may go in and dress it for me and my son, that we may eat it, and die. And Elijah said unto her, Fear not; go and do as thou hast said: but make me thereof a little cake first, and bring it unto me, and after make for thee and for thy son. For thus saith the Lord God of Israel, The barrel of meal shall not waste, neither shall the cruse of oil fail, until the day that the Lord sendeth rain upon the earth. And she went and did according to the saying of Elijah: and she, and he, and her house, did eat many days. And the barrel of meal wasted not, neither did the cruse of oil fail, according to the word of the Lord, which he spake by Elijah.

God fed, comforted, and restored Elijah in an unusual way. As he began to experience greater restoration, he was brought to this widow and depended upon her for further care, and in return this women and her son were blessed with abundance during a time of great famine in the land that God foretold through the prophet Elijah. In unexpected ways and means, God restored Elijah, the widow, and her son and a greater faith and trust in divine sustenance was learned. This is what all of us need at some time in our earthly journey. When illness comes, a greater dependence upon God is necessary in order experience complete wholeness! This rest is for you given as a blessing from God. "Come unto me, all ye that are weary and heavy laden, and I will give you rest."

Matthew Henry, a respected commentator on God's Word, defines this concept of rest:

> If Providence calls us to solitude and retirement, it becomes us to acquiesce; when we cannot be useful we must be patient, and when we cannot work for God we must sit still quietly for him. How he was fed. Though he could not work there, having nothing to do but to meditate and pray (which would help to prepare him for his usefulness afterwards), yet he shall eat, for he is in the way of his duty, and verily he shall be fed, in the day of famine he shall be satisfied. (Matthew Henry's Commentary on the Whole Bible).

Finally, realize that it is essential for you to know God on a personal level. Before you can understand His power, His grace, His rest, His sustenance fully, you must accept Him in your heart completely. Jesus said, "If ye abide in me, and my words abide in you, ye shall ask what ye will, and it shall be done unto you" (John 15:7). We must know that Jesus died so we may live. In order to know Him, we must denounce our old patterns of living, forsake our yesterdays, and accept His saving grace and become a follower of His way to the end of our human existence. His power is available for your healing. May God bless and heal you completely in body, soul, and spirit, and may your life be filled with peace, joy, and hope until His coming. Amen!

Chapter 15

Where the Rubber Meets the Road (Case Histories)

May God guide you, your loved ones, and your doctor to the appropriate, integrated treatment of cancer with the greatest result. Remission of cancer is the target and cure is the ultimate hope.

Il temp'e un gran medico. Time is a great healer.

—Italian Proverb

Where the rubber meets the road is when a cancer patient experiences remission from his or her cancer. *Remission* is the word that is frequently used to describe a cancer that is no longer active. The word *cure* means a cancer that has been totally healed. Yes, there are numerous accounts of people beating the odds of cancer. The following five cases are real experiences, but the names have been changed to protect privacy and confidentiality.

BREAST CANCER

Lisa is a fifty-year-old female who was diagnosed with breast cancer by her regular physician. She came to my office hoping that alternative medicine could help her. After much discussion, she decided to implement the suggested treatment plan. Fortunately, her cancer had not spread to other areas of her body. Her treatment plan consisted of the following:

- Intravenous immunotherapy (includes vitamins, minerals, amino acids, immune modulators)
- Autologous homeopathic vaccine
- C-Statin (an herbal formulation that discourages blood supply to tumor)
- MGN 3
- Beta 1,3-Glucan
- Larix
- CoQ10
- Selected Chinese botanicals
- Hoxsey formula
- B12, folic acid, and B comp injections one to two times weekly
- Multivitamin/mineral formula
- Adrenal support
- Rice protein support along with whole foods way of eating (food combining and alkaline/acid way of eating)
- Juicing
- Probiotics

Lisa also had several chemotherapy sessions, which consisted of Taxatera, Taxol, and Adriamycin. She is in complete remission.

LUNG CANCER WITH SPREAD TO THE BRAIN

Joanne, forty-five years old, came to my office after consulting many alternative practitioners. She was frustrated because she was on confusing regimens and feeling discouraged because her cancer was getting worse. Her diagnosis was lung cancer. She was having seizures when she came to see me. Joanne was a smoker and consumed moderate amounts of alcohol. She was told that she was going to die within the month because the cancer had spread to her brain and liver. I started Joanne on a comprehensive regimen and told her that she needed to work with an oncologist who was open to the alternatives. She agreed. I referred her to an oncologist with whom I work closely. The following regimen kept Joanne alive for three years:

- Intravenous immunotherapy (vitamins, minerals, amino acids, and immune modulators)

- MGN 3

- Beta 1,3-Glucan

- Larix

- Hoxsey formula

- CoQ10

- B12, folic acid, and B comp injections two times weekly

- Essiac formula

- Selected Chinese anti-tumor botanicals

- Dietary changes, which included cutting out red meats and juicing every day

- IP-6

- Several chemotherapy sessions (standard regimen for lung cancer)

The response to the regimen was excellent. After three months of therapy, we repeated an MRI to see if the cancer was clearing. MRI results demonstrated no brain lesions and liver metastasis was gone, and the size of the lung lesion that was previously grapefruit-size had shrunk to about the size of a golf ball. Joanne was so happy that she felt she didn't need to continue such a strict treatment regimen, and eventually her office visits became less frequent to none.

Joanne and I had an ongoing battle with her smoking. I told her that she needed to quit or the cancer would return. She didn't take the advice. About one year later, I received a call from Joanne, and she had a desperate tone. She said, "My cancer has returned! Can you please help me?" I told her I would. This time she stopped smoking. I put her on the same regimen and stepped up the frequency of her visits. Again, her cancer responded to treatment. But she began smoking again, and the cancer returned. She lived for three years, even though her doctors told her that she only had one month. This case makes me sad when I think of the many more years she could have had . . . if she had just stopped smoking.

PROSTATE CANCER

Dave is a sixty-year-old retired 747 captain . He is in great physical shape, except for the fact that he was just diagnosed with prostate cancer. He had a high PSA and a significant Gleason score. His biopsy demonstrated cancer confined to the prostate gland with no spread. He came to me by a referral, and he heard about the good things that were happening with the cancer patients I have had the opportunity to treat. I started him on a treatment regimen that consisted of:

- IP-6

- PC SPES (the FDA pulled this item because of high concentrations of Coumadin in the formulation)

- Beta 1,3-Glucan

- B12, folic acid, and B comp injections one to two times weekly

- CoQ10

- Vitamin E

- Concentrated Saw palmetto extract

- Multivitamin/mineral/antioxidant formula

- Dietary changes, which included intense juicing

Dave's PSA levels dramatically reduced to the normal range and allowed for the entrance into a treatment program that used proton therapy, rated a high cure rate for prostate cancer. We achieved excellent results with the alternative regimen, and Dave was happy. He wanted to be sure that the cancer was cured, so he enrolled in the proton treatment program at Loma Linda, and we continued supportive care. He made it through the treatment, and he is cancer-free and healthy!

MULTIPLE MYELOMA

Susan is a fifty-five-year-old female who came to see me after being diagnosed with multiple myeloma. She had heard the devastating stories of people who suffered with this form of cancer. She wanted to do everything she could from an alternative perspective that was safe and effective. She had one round of chemotherapy, and this made her very ill. She stopped and told me that she needed to do something naturally. I designed a program for her to follow:

- Beta 1, 3-Glucan

- MGN 3

- B12, folic acid, and B comp injections two times weekly

- Dietary changes, including juicing

- CoQ10

- Hoxsey formula

- Essiac formula

- Probiotics

- Selected Chinese botanicals with anti-tumor and immune modulating properties

- Immune enhancing therapy

- Creative stress management

Susan didn't need any more chemotherapy. She is currently in a steady state with no flare-up of the myeloma. This is going on five years from the time of the diagnosis. She is very happy to be alive and able to spend time with her loved ones, enjoying life.

BLADDER CANCER

James is a sixty-two-year-old male who came to the office with blood in his urine. An MRI demonstrated a visible tumor, and upon cystoscopic examination and biopsy, the tumor was diagnosed as being in its second stage. James was not too keen on chemotherapy and bladder removal. The recommendation of the urologist oncologist was to remove the bladder totally. James took the proactive approach and searched out his therapy. He came to me for answers and we provided these answers. James began our natural cancer treatment program, and we worked together with an oncologist to search out the best conventional therapy. His program included several radiation treatments and low dose Gemcitabine to sensitize the cancer cells to the radiation, along with his natural medicine protocol and autologous vaccine. In six months the tumor was completely gone, confirmed on cystoscopy and biopsy. James came in for IV immune support therapy twice weekly. He continues today to be cancer free. One of the most essential aspects of James and his healing experience is that we prayed earnestly for his healing and recovery consistently.

There are many more cases like these that include lymphoma, leukemia, testicular cancer, and sarcomas. The common theme of all these cases is that life was extended and the quality of life improved. In addition, there is even the hope of being cured. There is also another vital element in all of these cases that I must tell you about, and that is prayer. In every case that comes, I pray for guidance and prudence in developing a plan. In addition, I petition God on my patient's behalf, asking that He would cause the cancer to remit and, if it is His will, to be cured. I mention specifically that cancer cells with their genetic traits would die and healthy cells would develop, free from all cancer. In my opinion, the credit for the healing in these cases belongs to God! May He also guide you, your loved ones, and your doctor to the best, integrated approach to cancer with the greatest result.

Chapter **16**

● ●

Conclusions and Cancer Resources

Integrating the best treatment options available is the key to healing. Some treatments are known to be curative and some are experimental. It is necessary to be informed as to the treatments available and when to integrate treatments.

This book is compiled to give you, the health-conscious individual, more information so you can make a better health care choice. When it comes to cancer, you need to know. God bless your healing journey.

TESTING RESOURCES

AMAS ONCOLAB, 36 The Fenway, Boston, MA 02215. 1.800.922.8378

CBC: Carbon Based Corporation. 1.702.832.8485

ELISA/ACT: Formerly Serammune Physicians Lab. 1.800.553.5472

ION and Oxidative Protection Panel: MetaMetrix, Inc., 5000 Peachtree Ind. Blvd., Norcross, GA 30071.

1.800.221.4640;
www.metametrix.com

ImmunoSciences Laboratory
www.immuno-sci-lab.com
E-mail: immunsci@ix.netcom.com
Phone: (310) 657-1077
Fax: (310) 657-1053
Toll Free: (800) 950-4686

NATIONAL CANCER INSTITUTE INFORMATION RESOURCES

Cancer Information Service (CIS)

You may want more information for yourself, your family, and your doctor. The following National Cancer Institute (NCI) services are available to help you. They provide accurate, up-to-date information on cancer to patients and their families, health professionals, and the general public. Information specialists translate the latest scientific information into understandable language and respond in English, Spanish, or on TTY equipment. Toll-free: 1.800.4-CANCER (1.800.422.6237) TTY: 1.800.332.8615

INTERNET INFORMATION

Health&Wellness Institute ®
5603 230th St. S.W.
Mountlake Terrace, WA 98043
1.425.697.6112
www.ehealthandhealing.com

American Cancer Society
1599 Clifton Road, N.E.
Atlanta, GA 30329-4251

1.800.ACS.2345
www.cancer.org

Cancer Research Institute
681 Fifth Avenue
New York, NY 10022-4209
1.800.33.CANCER
www.cancerresearch.org

Cancer Care, Inc.
1180 Avenue of the Americas
New York, NY 10036
1.800.813.HOPE
www.cancercareinc.org

The Candlelighters Childhood Cancer Foundation
7910 Woodmont Ave., #460
Bethesda, MD 20814-3015
1.800.366.2223
www.candlelighters.org

Cancer Research Foundation of America
200 Daingerfield Road, #200
Alexandria, VA 22314
1.800.227.CRFA
www.preventcancer.org

National Cancer Institute
31 Center Drive/MSC 2580
Building 31, Room 10A07
Bethesda, MD 20892-2580
1.800.4.CANCER
www.nci.nih.gov

National Comprehensive Cancer Network (NCCN)
This web site has alliance members listed. Each one is a leading cancer center. The listing is complete and the web address below will assist you further.
www.nccn.org

NATUROPATHIC PHYSICIAN ASSOCIATION (REFERRALS)

www.naturopathic.org
1.877.969.2267

WORK AND CAREER RELATED ISSUES FOR CANCER PATIENTS

Equal Employment Opportunity Commission
www.eeoc.gov
www.cancerandcareers.org

ADDITIONAL INTERNET SITES

www.cancerhelp.net
www.searchforcures.com
www.phrma.org (listing of the latest cancer research drugs)
www.cancermed.com
www.issels.com
www.cancerandcareers.org
www.cancernet.nci.nih.gov
www.chelation.com
www.metametrix.com
www.llu.edu
www.cancersource.com

Appendix 1

• •

Common Chemotherapeutic and Biological Agents

Alkylating Agents and Platinum Compounds

Alkylating agents and platinum compounds cause damage to the cell's DNA structure. These agents are extremely toxic to the cells of every system of the body. Nerve damage, heart damage, and other organ damage is not uncommon when using these agents. If considering this as part of treatment, then I recommend an integrative treatment program. A sample of this is listed in Appendices 3, 4, 5, and 6. It is essential that you consult with your physician specializing in integrative cancer medicine. Other adverse effects include nausea, vomiting, fatigue, and mouth ulcers.

Altretamine-Paraplatin)(Hexalen)
BCNU- (Carmustine)
Busulfan- (Myleran)
Chlorambucil- (Leukeran)
Cyclophosphamide- (Cytoxan)
Fotemustine- (Muphoran)
Iphosphamide- (Ifex)
Iomustine- (CCNU)

Melphalan- (Alkeran)
Nitrogen mustard- (Mustargen)
Pipobroman- (Vercyte)
Procarbazine- (Matulane)
Streptozocin- (Zanosar)
Streptozotocin- (Zanosar)
Temozolomide- (Temodar)
Thiotepa- (Thioplex)

Triethylenemelamine- (TEM)

Carboplatin- (Paraplatin)
Cisplatin- (Platinol)

293

Anti-tumor Antibiotics

Antibiotics that have tumor fighting properties are known as anti-tumor antibiotics. The action of these antibiotics is on DNA, by interfering with synthesis or with processes that are controlled by DNA signals. A broad variety of cancers are treated with anti-tumor antibiotics. The most common side reaction is anemia caused by bone marrow suppression. The heart can also be harmed, which can be life threatening. Other adverse effects include nausea, vomiting, fatigue, and mouth ulcers.

Actinomycin-D- (Cosmegen)   Epirubicin- (Ellence)
Bleomycin sulfate- (Blenoxane)   Idarubicin- (Idamycin)
Daunomycin- (Cerubidine)   Mitomycin-C- (Mutamycin)
Daunorubicin- (Cerubidine)   Mitramycin- (Mithracin)
Doxorubicin- (Adriamycin, Doxil)

Appendix 1 (cont'd)
Common Chemotherapeutic and Biological Agents

Anti-metabolites

Anti-metabolites interfere with the production of genetic material (DNA and RNA) in the cell. These agents are less toxic to the cells as compared to other chemotherapy agents. They are often combined with other chemotherapy agents. Adverse effects include anemia, nausea, vomiting, diarrhea, hair loss, and fatigue. See Appendix 6 for oral supplementation to help with some of these side effects. In cases where Methotrexate (MTX) is used, large doses of folic acid need to be avoided; 400-800 mcg of folic acid is safe in combination with MTX and will not impair the action of the drug. Nutrient support is essential, particularly protein, because protein metabolism is affected by the drug. Protein supplementation in the form of rice and/or whey, approximately 25 grams twice daily, is recommended.

Asparaginase- (Elspar)	Fluorouracil- (5-FU)
Chlorodeoxyadenosine- (Leustatin)	Gemcitabine- (Gemzar)
Cytosine arabinoside- (Ara-C,	Hydroxyurea- (Hydrea)
Cytosar-U)	Mercaptopurine- (6-MP)
Deoxycoformycin- (Nipent)	Methotrexate- (Folex, MTX)
Floxuridine- (5-FUDR)	Thioguanine- (6-TG)
Fludarabine phosphate- (Fludara)	

Biological Response Modifiers

Biological response modifiers are compounds that modulate the immune system and how it reacts to cancer. Interferons and Interleukins are examples that work directly by slowing cancer cell growth. Toxic effects include flu-like symptoms, fatigue, headache, joint pain, and muscle aches. These drugs are usually very expensive and are considered along with other chemotherapy agents in combination or as single agents.

Alpha Interferon- (Intron A, Roferon-A)
Bacillus Calmette-Guerin- (BCG)
Erythropoietin- (EPO, Epogen)
G-CSF- (Neupogen)
GM-CSF- (Leukine, Prokine)
Interleukin-2- (Proleukin, Aldesleukin)
Interleukin12

Appendix 1 (cont'd)
Common Chemotherapeutic and
Biological Agents

Hormones and Hormone Inhibitors

Hormones are chemical agents in the body that are produced by certain organs to initiate, facilitate, or inhibit certain function in organs and systems of the body. With cancer some tumors respond to the presence of hormones. Tumor activity can be altered negatively by the presence of hormones in favor of cancer cell growth or favorably to inhibit cancer cell growth. See Appendix 6 for an oral supplementation plan that can assist with the negative reactions associated with these agents.

ADVERSE REACTIONS:

- Hormonal agents are generally well tolerated and usually don't produce severe side reactions.
- Anti-hormonal agents have common side effects that include nausea, vomiting, indigestion, and hot flashes. Bone marrow suppression, which can lead to anemia, usually disappears as treatment resumes.
- Anti-estrogen agents can cause headaches, flaking and brittle fingernails, visual disturbance and endometrial changes including *endometrial cancer. Soy products should be avoided when taking the drug Tamoxifen, and soy foods should be limited to no more than five servings per week.*
- Microtubule Inhibitors and Chromatin Inhibitors can cause nausea, diarrhea, mouth sores, anemia fever, chills, skin rash, and allergic reactions.
- Molecular Targeted Agents cause very few known side effects. These agents are relatively new, and ongoing research is necessary to establish efficacy and safety. These agents demonstrate favorable results in specific cancers. *See more information on Gleevec, Herceptin, and Rituxin in chapter seven.*

Common Chemotherapeutic and Biological Agents

CORTICOSTEROIDS

- Betamethasone sodium phosphate (Celestone phosphate)
- Cortisone acetate (Cortisone)
- Dexamethasone (Decadron)
- Dexamethasone acetate (Dalalone D.P.)
- Hydrocortisone (Hydrocortone)
- Prednisolone (Prelone)
- Prednisilone tebutate (Hydeltra-TBA)

ANTICORTICOSTEROID

- Estrogens (DES, Estrace, Premarin, Estatab, Orthoest, EstroSpan, Valegren)
- Progestins (Depo-Provera)
- Antiestrogens (Arimidex-anastrozole, Femera-letrozole, Evista-raloxifene, Nolvadex-tamoxifen)
- Estrogen/Progesterone combinations (Prempro)

Common Chemotherapy Regimens in Cancer Treatment

(COMBINATION AND SINGLE AGENT REGIMENS)

The following is a valuable resource in understanding in greater detail current chemotherapy regimens as the most common treatments in cancer. These treatments vary, depending upon the oncologist. Oncologists have their special regimens and may prefer other agents. Having the knowledge of what regimens are currently used can assist you in speaking with the oncologists about alternatives. Below you will find a sample of this valuable reference.

Physicians' Cancer Chemotherapy Drug Manual 2002 Monograph
For more information: **www.jbpub.com** or **info@jbpub.com** or **www.cancersource.com**

Generic Drug Name: Doxorubicin
Trade names: Adriamycin, Adria, Hydroxydaunorubicin, DOX, Rubex
Classification: Anti-tumor antibiotic
Category: Chemotherapy drug
Drug manufacturer: Pharmacia

Mechanism of action:

- Anthracycline antibiotic isolated from *Streptomyces* species

- Intercalates into DNA, resulting in inhibition of DNA synthesis and function

- Inhibits transcription through inhibition of DNA-dependent RNA polymerase

- Inhibits topoisomerase II by forming a cleavable complex with DNA and topoisomerase II to create uncompensated DNA helix torsional tension, leading to eventual DNA breaks

- Formation of cytotoxic oxygen-free radicals results in single- and double-stranded DNA breaks with subsequent inhibition of DNA synthesis and function

Mechanism of resistance:

- Increased expression of the multidrug-resistant gene with elevated P170 levels. This leads to increased drug efflux and decreased intracellular drug accumulation.

- Decreased expression of topoisomerase II.

- Mutation in topoisomerase II with decreased binding affinity to doxorubicin.

- Increased expression of sulfhydryl proteins, including glutathione and glutathione-dependent proteins.

Absorption: Not absorbed orally.

Distribution: Widely distributed to tissues. Does not cross the blood-brain barrier. About 75% of doxorubicin and its metabolites are bound to plasma proteins.

Metabolism: Metabolized extensively in the liver to the active hydroxylated metabolite, doxorubicinol. About 40–50% of drug is eliminated via biliary excretion in feces. Less than 10% of the drug is cleared by the kidneys. Prolonged terminal half-life of twenty to forty-eight hours.

Indications:

1. Breast cancer

2. Hodgkin's and non-Hodgkin's lymphoma

3. Soft tissue sarcoma

4. Ovarian cancer

5. Non–small cell and small cell lung cancer

6. Bladder cancer

7. Thyroid cancer

8. Hepatoma

9. Gastric cancer

10. Wilms' tumor

11. Neuroblastoma

12. Acute lymphoblastic leukemia

Dosage range:

1. Single agent: 60–75 mg/m^2 IV every three weeks

2. Single agent: 15–20 mg/m^2 IV weekly

3. Combination therapy: 45–60 mg/m^2 every three weeks

4. Continuous infusion: 60–90 mg/m^2 IV over ninety-six hours

Drug preparation:

- Available in 10, 20, 50, 100, and 150 mg vials for IV use. Also available in 200 mg multidose vial.

- Dilute with 0.9% sodium chloride (preservative-free) to yield a final concentration of 2 mg/ml. May be further diluted in 0.9% sodium chloride for prolonged infusions.

- Reconstituted solution is stable for seven days at room temperature and for fifteen days under refrigeration.

- Doxorubicin is compatible in solution with vincristine in prolonged infusions.

Drug interaction:

- Drug interaction 1: Dexamethasone, 5-FU, heparin—Doxorubicin is incompatible with dexamethasone, 5-FU, and heparin, as concurrent use will lead to precipitate formation.

- Drug interaction 2: Dexrazoxane—The cardiotoxic effects of doxorubicin are inhibited by the iron-chelating agent dexrazoxane (ICRF-187, Zinecard).

- Drug interaction 3: Cyclophosphamide—Increased risk of hemorrhagic cystitis and cardiotoxicity when doxorubicin is given with cyclophosphamide. Important to be able to distinguish between hemorrhagic cystitis and the normal red-orange urine observed with doxorubicin therapy.

- Drug interaction 4: Phenobarbital, phenytoin—Increased plasma clearance of doxorubicin when given concurrently with barbiturates and phenytoin.

- Drug interaction 5: Herceptin, mitomycin-C—Increased risk of cardiotoxicity when doxorubicin is given with herceptin or mitomycin-C.

- Drug interaction 6: Digoxin—Doxorubicin decreases the oral bioavailability of digoxin.

- Drug interaction 7: 6-Mercaptopurine—Increased risk of hepatotoxicity when doxorubicin is given with 6-mercaptopurine.

Special considerations:

1. Use with caution in patients with abnormal liver function. Dose reduction is required in the setting of liver dysfunction.

2. Because doxorubicin is a strong vesicant, administer slowly with a rapidly flowing IV. Avoid using veins over joints or in extremities with compromised venous and/or lymphatic drainage.

3. Use of a central venous catheter is recommended for patients with difficult venous access and mandatory for prolonged infusions.

4. Careful monitoring is necessary to avoid extravasation. If extravasation is suspected, immediately stop infusion, withdraw fluid, elevate extremity, and apply ice to involved site. May administer local steroids. In severe cases, consult a plastic surgeon.

5. Monitor cardiac function before (baseline) and periodically during therapy with either MUGA radionuclide scan or echocardiogram to assess LVEF. Risk of cardiotoxicity is higher in patients > 70 years of age, in patients with prior history of hypertension or preexisting heart disease, in patients previously treated with anthracyclines, or in patients with prior radiation therapy to the chest. Cumulative doses of > 550 mg/m^2 are associated with increased risk for cardiotoxicity.

6. Risk of cardiotoxicity is decreased with weekly or continuous infusion schedules. Use of the iron-chelating

agent dexrazoxane (ICRF-187) also is effective at reducing the development of cardiotoxicity.

7. Use with caution in patients previously treated with radiation therapy as doxorubicin can cause radiation recall skin reaction. Increased risk of skin toxicity when doxorubicin is given concurrently with radiation therapy.

8. Patients should be cautioned to avoid sun exposure and to wear sun protection when outside.

9. Patients should be warned about the potential for red-orange discoloration of urine for one to two days after drug administration.

10. Pregnancy category D. Breast-feeding should be avoided.

Toxicity

- Toxicity 1: Myelosuppression. Dose-limiting toxicity with leukopenia more common than thrombocytopenia or anemia. Nadir usually occurs at days ten through fourteen with full recovery by day twenty-one.

- Toxicity 2: Nausea and vomiting. Usually mild, occurring in 50% of patients within the first one to two hours of treatment.

- Toxicity 3: Mucositis and diarrhea. Common but not dose-limiting.

- Toxicity 4: Cardiotoxicity. Acute form presents within the first two to three days as arrhythmias and/or conduction abnormalities, EKG changes, pericarditis, and/or myocarditis. Usually transient and mostly asymptomatic. Not dose-related. Chronic form results in a dose-dependent, dilated cardiomyopathy associated with congestive heart failure. Risk increases when cumulative doses are greater than 550 mg/m^2.

- Toxicity 5: Strong vesicant. Extravasation can lead to tissue necrosis and chemical thrombophlebitis at the site of injection.

- Toxicity 6: Hyperpigmentation of nails, rarely skin rash, and urticaria. Radiation recall skin reaction can occur at prior sites of irradiation. Increased hypersensitivity to sunlight.

- Toxicity 7: Alopecia. Universal but usually reversible within three months after termination of treatment.

- Toxicity 8: Red-orange discoloration of urine. Usually occurs within one to two days after drug administration.

- Toxicity 9: Allergic, hypersensitivity reactions are rare.

Chemotherapy Agents Listed In Book:

Aldesleukin
Alemtuzumab
Altretamine
Amifostine
Aminoglutethimide
Amsacrine
Anastrozole
Arsenic trioxide
Asparaginase

Bacillus Calmette-Guérin (BCG)
Bexarotene
Bicalutamide

Bleomycin
Buserelin
Busulfan

Capecitabine
Carboplatin
Carmustine
Chlorambucil
Cisplatin
Cladribine
Cyclophosphamide
Cytarabine

Dactinomycin-D
Daunorubicin
Daunorubicin liposome

Denileukin diftitox
Dexamethasone
Dexrazoxane
Diphenhydramine
Docetaxel
Dolasetron
Doxorubicin
Doxorubicin (liposome)
Dronabinol

Erythropoietin
Estramustine
Etoposide
Etoposide phosphate
Exemestane

Filgrastim
Floxuridine
Fludarabine
5-Fluorouracil
Flutamide

Gemcitabine
Gemtuzumab (ozo-gamicin)
Goserelin
Granisetron

Hydroxyurea

Idarubicin
Ifosfamide
Imatinib
Interferon-?
Irinotecan
Isotretinoin

Letrozole
Leucovorin
Leuprolide
Lomustine
Lorazepam

Mechlorethamine
Megestrol acetate
Melphalan
Mercaptopurine
Mesna
Methotrexate
Metoclopramide
Mitomycin-C
Mitotane
Mitoxantrone

Nilutamide

Ondansetron
Oxaliplatin

Paclitaxel
Pemetrexed
Pentostatin
Procarbazine
Prochlorperazine

Raltitrexed
Rituximab

Sargramostim
Streptozocin
Tamoxifen
Temozolomide
Teniposide

Thalidomide
Thiethylperazine
Thioguanine
Thiotepa
Topotecan
Toremifene
Trastuzumab
Tretinoin
Trimetrexate

UFT

Vinblastine
Vincristine
Vinorelbine

Sample Nutritional Intravenous (IV) Cancer Protocol

IV TREATMENT PROTOCOL (IV THERAPY ONE TO TWO TIMES WEEKLY)

- Folate (contraindicated with some chemotherapeutic agents)
- Germanium sesquioxide
- Calcium gluconate
- Chromium
- Glycyrrhizic acid (contraindicated in hypertension)
- Magnesium sulfate
- Molybdenum
- MSM
- MTE 5 minerals (concentrated)
- Potassium chloride

- Saline 0.9%

- Super B-Comp (European source)

- Vitamin B12

- Zinc chloride

- Modified Issine Formula (AN-1) 2–3ml (proprietary formulation)

IV therapy is designed to enhance immune function and give general nutritional replacement. It is useful in chronic illness, cancer, and nutritional deficiencies. Vitamin C can be administered after the main nutrient IV. Vitamin C and trace minerals should be put together due to oxidation reaction.

Appendix 4

Sample Injection Cancer
Treatment Protocol

1. CoQ10 IM at 1–1.5 ml in hip one to three times weekly

2. Thymus Peptide 1ml IM one to three times weekly

3. Lipoic Acid 1ml IM one to three times weekly

4. Some additional homeopathics: Placenta compositium and Viscum compositum. (Iscador)

Each treatment plan varies with individual patients and depends upon their clinical need and tolerance to therapy.

Appendix 5

Artemesia Treatment Protocol

Artemisinin: A lipid soluble form of Artemesia annua

Dose: One to two mg/kg of body weight

Timing: In the evening, *four* hours after last meal, with a small amount of water or milk, only (not with food due to iron content)

Administration: By mouth to start, with two test doses and then evaluate

Duration: Six weeks and then evaluate with labs

Drug interactions: none known

Product name: Hepalin

Artesunate: A water-soluble form of Artemesia annua

Dose: 0.5-1 mg/kg of body weight

Timing: One injection/day (preferably in the evening)

Administration: Dissolve 60 mg in one ml of sodium bicarbonate, shake for two to three minutes until the mixture becomes clear. Make sure to do this out of direct light as much as possible. Add 2 ml of normal saline. Mix well, and fill syringe. Inject I.M.; two test doses and then evaluate

Duration: Six weeks and then evaluate with labs

Drug interactions: none known

Artemix: A combination of Artemisinin, Artesunate, and Artemeter (oral form)

Lactoferrin: 250 mg, two times per day. (Used to bind iron.) Do not give lactoferrin at the same time as artemesia because it can inhibit the effectiveness of the artemesia. Take the lactoferrin during the day-time.

Vitamin C: 500 mg BID away from meals, morning, and around lunch-time

Contraindications: Do not take any artemesia products within four weeks of radiation treatment.

Test recommendations:

MRI

- In cases of brain tumors, establish a baseline MRI. After six weeks of therapy, do another MRI.

Blood Work

- CBC—to evaluate levels of anemia and immune function
- Tumor markers: to evaluate tumor progression

Sample Natural Cancer Treatment Plan (Chemotherapy and Radiation Therapy)

ORAL REGIMEN

- Protease enzymes dosage recommendations by your physicians fifteen to twenty minutes before meals.

- Quercetin—800 mg daily, fifteen to twenty minutes away from food, not on the same day of chemotherapy and radiation therapy. With chemotherapy, curcumin is recommended.

- General oncological support vitamin/mineral combination based upon body weight and individual need. Can be taken at any time and will not interfere with chemotherapy or radiation therapy.

- Vitamin C—2000 mg three times daily, not on the same day of chemotherapy or radiation therapy.

- Vitamin E—800 IU daily, not on the same day of chemotherapy or radiation therapy.

- Probiotics—one-half teaspoon non-dairy source, two times a day.

- Green Tea Extract—600-800 mg daily, not on the same day of chemotherapy or radiation therapy.

- Vitamin B6—150 mg daily.

- CoQ10—400-600 mg daily, not on the same day of chemotherapy or radiation therapy.

- Folic acid—400-800 mcg daily.

- Maitake fractions—1mg daily for every 2.2 pounds of body weight or PSP/PSK 3000 mg daily, away from food.

- Indole-3-Carbinol (beneficial in all cancers)—500 mg daily.

- C-Statin and ImmKine for tumor regression and immune support.

One week prior to beginning radiation start 15,000 IU of vitamin A (can be in the form of cod liver oil and beta-carotene 125 mg daily).

Mouth Sores

For mouth sores: DGL (licorice) Sorbic wash and probiotic powder as an oral tonic during conventional treatment. In addition, Jason Cosmetic CoQ10 tooth gel and Young Living Essential Oil Dentarome Plus tooth gel can be restorative and healing because they contain essential oils, CoQ10, and Coenzyme A as well as healing botanicals.

Other botanicals may be preferred by your physician. The above are recommendations to consider and doesn't take the place of prescribed medical treatment.

This above protocol should be supported with IV nutritional immune therapy

Glossary

2'-Deoxycoformycin—(see pentostatin).

5-Fluorouracil—Also known as 5-FU, an anti-metabolite class of chemotherapy drug.

5-FUDR—(see floxuridine).

6-MP—(see mercaptopurine).

6-TG.—(see thioguanine).

Ablative oophorectomy—Surgery that renders the ovaries inactive.

ABVD—A combination of the chemotherapy drugs doxorubicin, bleomycin, vinblastine, and dacarbazine.

Acupuncture—A branch of oriental medicine that involves the use of needles, electrical voltage, or pressure to stimulate "meridians of energy flow" in the body.

Adaptogen—A substance, usually an herb, that is thought to normalize human functions.

Adenopathy—Swelling of lymph glands.

Adrenal Cortical Carcinoma—Cancer of the adrenal gland.

Adriamycin—(see doxorubicin).

Aflatoxin—A fungus found on certain edible plants, including peanuts, which can cause liver cancer.

Aldesleukin—Also known as interleukin, this is a biological agent chemotherapy drug.

Alkaloids—Medicinal ingredients found in herbs and other plants.

Alkylating agents—A class of chemotherapy drugs that attacks cancer by creating substances known as free radicals.

Allergy—An immune response to an allergen. Allergens are numerous and can include foods, pollen, chemicals, dust, fibers, and many other substances. Different individuals can have allergies to different allergens.

Allogeneic transplant—Using someone else's cells for a bone marrow transplant. (See also bone marrow transplant.)

Altretamine—Also known as Hexamethylmelamine, this is an alkylating agent class of chemotherapy drug.

Amino acids—The chemical building blocks that make up a complete protein. There are nine essential amino acids that must be in the diet since they cannot be synthesized by the body as well as thirteen nonessential amino acids, which can be synthesized by the body.

Aminoglutethimide—Also known as Cytadren, this is a hormonal class of chemotherapy drug.

Amitriptyline—A tricyclic anti-depressant drug that is sometimes used to treat cancer pain.

Analgesic—A type of painkiller that includes both drugs and herbs.

Anemia—A condition in which the blood has too few red cells and/or reduced hemoglobin. Anemia can result in reduced ability to carry oxygen from the lungs to the tissues needing it. Symptoms can include fatigue and pale skin.

Anthracyclines—A subclass within the anti-tumor antibiotic class of chemotherapy drugs.

Antibiotic—A drug that helps to eliminate agents such as bacteria, viruses, and funguses that can cause infection.

Antibody—A protein in the body usually developed by the immune system to respond to and destroy a particular foreign substance or antigen.

Anticonvulsant—A drug that relieves or prevents convulsions.

Antidepressant—A drug for the relief of depression. Subclasses of antidepressants include selective serotonin re-uptake inhibitors (SSRI), monoamine oxidase inhibitors (MAOI), and tricyclics.

Antigen—Any substance, usually foreign to the body, that evokes a defense response from the immune system. Antigens can include chemicals, foods, bacteria, and toxins.

Antimetabolite—A class of chemotherapy drugs that interferes with the metabolism and reproduction of tumor cells.

Antineoplastic agents—Drugs that inhibit or prevent the development of tumor cells. Chemotherapy drugs are antineoplastic agents.

Antioxidant—A substance that quenches free radicals in the body. A free radical that has been quenched by antioxidants is no longer capable of damaging cells in the body. Antioxidants include certain vitamins, minerals, herbs, and other substances.

Antipsychotic—A class of drugs used for the treatment of psychiatric disorders.

Anti-tumor antibiotic—A class of chemotherapy drugs whose chemical structure resembles traditional antibiotics. Like alkylating agents, most anti-tumor antibiotics create free radicals that attack rapidly dividing tumor cells.

Apoptosis—Programmed cell death. Apoptosis is a very popular term in cancer therapy and has a strong relationship in influencing the genetics of cancer.

Arginine—A non-essential amino acid.

Ascorbic acid—Known as Vitamin C and is very effective vitamin in cancer treatment.

Asparaginase—An enzyme that breaks down the nonessential amino acid asparagines. Asparaginase is also a drug known as L-asparaginase or ELSPAR, which is an antimetabolite class of chemotherapy drug.

Astrocytoma—A tumor of the nervous system, which includes the brain.

Autologous transplant—Using the patient's own cells for transplant.

Autologous vaccine—A vaccine that is made from a patient's own serum and processed with biological agents such as IL-12, Interferon and polypeptides.

Bacillus Calmette-Guerin (BCG)—A biological agent class of chemotherapy drug. It is a live bacterial strain that is administered directly to the site of certain urinary tract cancers.

BCNU—(see carmustine).

Beta-carotene—The precursor to vitamin A.

BFM—An intensive combination of chemotherapy drugs used for the treatment of leukemia.

BiCNU—(see carmustine).

Biliary system—A system of tubes connecting the liver and pancreas to the small intestine. Bile from the liver as well as pancreatic enzymes flow through these tubes to the small intestine, providing digestive enzymes as well as eliminating toxins. The biliary system also includes the gall bladder, which stores bile until needed.

Bioflavonoid—Also known as vitamin P, these are yellow pigments found in fruits, vegetables, and grains. Nearly 1,000 varieties have been identified. They have not been shown to be essential in human nutrition but do improve the function of vitamin C and suggested anticancer activity.

Biological agent—A class of chemotherapy drugs that are living organisms or act like parts of living organisms such as chemicals normally found in the body.

Biopsy—Procedure for obtaining a tissue sample for analysis and diagnosis.

Bleomycin—An anti-tumor antibiotic chemotherapy drug.

Blood chemistries—Blood tests that examine a variety of enzymes, hormones, and other chemicals.

Bone marrow—The cells inside bones that manufacture many but not all the cells of the immune system and blood.

Bone marrow suppression—Reduction of the ability of the bone marrow to produce adequate white blood cells and/or red blood cells and/or platelets. In some cases, suppressed marrow may produce adequate numbers of cells but with cells that do not perform properly.

Bone marrow transplant—The process of eliminating the existing bone marrow with very high dose conventional cancer treatments such as chemotherapy and/or radiation and replacing with bone marrow from the patient (autologous) or from another person (allogeneic). Bone marrow damage may be secondary to treatment or purposeful to eliminate defective marrow function.

Brachytherapy—The process of implanting radioactive "seeds" within or very close to a tumor. The seeds release a slow, steady dose of radiation. Brachytherapy has the advantage of being very specific and localized, thereby, reducing damage to healthy tissue.

Burkitt's Lymphoma—A type of lymph system cancer.

Busulfan—An alkylating agent chemotherapy drug.

Camptothecan—(see irinotecan).

Cannabinoid—A drug or substance that acts like cannabis, such as marijuana.

Carboplatin—An alkylating agent chemotherapy drug.

Carcinogen—A substance that can cause cancer.

Carcinoid—A hormone-producing cancer.

Carcinoid syndrome—A condition caused by carcinoid tumors that includes hot flashes, diarrhea, breathing difficulty, and heart problems.

Carcinoid tumor—A cancerous tumor that secretes hormones. When the tumor is located on the liver or a vulnerable part of the digestive system or some other rare site, the secreted hormones can create carcinoid syndrome.

Carcinomatosis—The condition of widespread cancer throughout the body.

Cardiac toxicity—Damage to the heart.

Carmustine—Also known as BCNU, an alkylating agent chemotherapy drug.

CAT scan—(see computerized axial tomography).

Central Nervous System (CNS)—The brain and spinal cord and the nerves that emanate from them. Also known as CNS.

Cerubidine—(see daunorubicin).

Chelation therapy—The use of drugs in the blood that bind to and remove unwanted substances. Most commonly used with the drug EDTA (ethylenediamine-tetraacetic acid) to remove plaque from the arteries of patients with cardiovascular disease.

Chemoprevention—The use of dietary and other substances to prevent cancer.

Chemoradiotherapy—The combination of chemotherapy and radiation at the same time, used usually for the purpose of intensifying the actions of both.

Chemotherapy—The use of any chemical to treat any disease. The term has been used more narrowly to describe drugs used for the treatment of cancer.

Chiropractors—Practitioners providing chiropractic adjustment, a form of manipulation of the spine.

Chlorambucil—An alkylating agent chemotherapy drug.

CHOP—A chemotherapy drug combination.

Cisplatin—Also known as Platinol, an alkylating agent chemotherapy drug.

Cladribine—An antimetabolite class of chemotherapy agent.

Clear margin—When a tumor can be removed with a measurable margin of tissue that has no visible cancer. Clear margin usually means the entire tumor has been removed.

Codeine—A pain-killer drug. An analgesic.

Cognition—Awareness of surroundings, perception, and memory.

Colonoscopy—A diagnostic screening procedure that visually inspects the inside of the colon. A biopsy can be taken during this procedure to assess abnormal tissue such as polyps.

Colony Stimulating Factors (CSF)—Drugs that mimic naturally occurring chemicals in the body that stimulate bone marrow manufacturing of certain cells.

Colostomy—Surgery to make the bowel exit the body into an appliance rather than the anus.

Complementary medicine—Combining conventional medicine with alternative medicine.

pproach

Computerized Axial Tomography—Radiographic technique that provides a three-dimensional view of the body and its internal parts.

Constipation—Bowel movements that are infrequent, hard, or require straining for elimination.

Cushing's syndrome—The result of excess secretion of the adrenal glands or high doses of corticosteroid drugs such as prednisone. Symptoms include puffiness, fatigue, weakness, loss of periods, and sometimes other symptoms, depending on dose and condition.

CVP—A chemotherapy drug combination.

Cyclophosphamide—Also known as Cytoxan, an alkylating agent chemotherapy drug.

Cystitis—An infection or inflammation of the urinary bladder.

Cytadren—(see aminoglutethimide).

Cytarabine—An antimetabolite class of chemotherapy drug.

Cytosine Arabinoside—(see cyarabine).

Cytotoxic—Capable of killing cells. In the case of cancer treatment, capable of killing cancer cells.

Dacarbazine—Also known as DTIC, an alkylating agent chemotherapy drug.

Dactinomycin—An anti-tumor antibiotic class of chemotherapy drug.

Daily Recommended —Also known as Daily Value, DRV, and DV, this is the level of oral nutrients such as vitamins and minerals recommended by the US Food and Drug Administration. These replace the recommended Daily Allowance, or RDA.

Daunorubicin—Also known as Cerubidine, an anti-tumor antibiotic class of chemotherapy agent.

DCF—(see Pentostatin).

Debulking—Process by which size of a tumor is reduced prior to surgery. Debulking usually involves chemotherapy or radiation.

Dementia—Term used to describe the general loss of mental function including memory, judgment, abstract reasoning, and personality.

DES—(see diethylstilbestrol).

Dexamethasone—Also known as Decadron, a steroid drug with many uses including controlling swelling and pressure from brain tumors.

DHAP—A chemotherapy drug combination.

Diabetes—A disease marked by inability to control blood sugar (glucose), inadequate insulin production or utilization, and excessive urination.

Diarrhea—Stool that is watery or very frequent.

Dietary fiber—Dietary fiber includes soluble and insoluble fiber.

Diethylstilbestrol—Synthetic estrogen, also known as DES.

Dilantin—Anticonvulsion drug. Often used in when brain tumors to control convulsive activity.

Docetaxel—Also known as Taxotere, a plant-derived class of chemotherapy drug. Often used as a alternative to Taxol.

Doxorubicin—Also known as Adriamycin, an anti-tumor antibiotic class of chemotherapy agent.

Edema—Retention of fluid, which causes puffiness. Can be side effect of some medications.

Effusion—Fluid into part of the body where fluid is not ordinary found.

Electromagnetic Field (EMF)—The electrical field that surrounds power lines and house wiring. It has been known to cause certain cancers.

Extreme Low Frequency (ELF)—Electromagnetic fields can emit low frequency.

Encephalopathy—A disease of the brain that may cause brain swelling.

Endocrine—This is the hormonal system of the human body.

Endometrium—The inside lining of the uterus.

Engraftment—The process of bone marrow transplantation that facilitates new blood cells to form.

Enteral—Pertaining to the small intestine.

Enzyme—Usually a protein that facilitates a reaction in the body without being changed itself.

Epirubicin—An anti-tumor antibiotic class of chemotherapy.

Epithelium—Layer of cells found on the surface of the skin, organs, and blood vessels.

Evening Primrose Oil (EPO)—An essential fatty acid.

Epoietin (EPO)—A hormone that stimulates the growth of red blood cells.

Epstein-Barr Virus (EBV)—A virus associated with mononucleosis, chronic fatigue, Burkitt's lymphoma, and nasopharyngeal carcinoma.

Esophagus—The part of the body that carries food from the mouth to the stomach. It is a hollow tube that is part of the digestive process.

Essential fatty acids—These are oils needed by the body for certain biochemical process and must be attained by the diet because they are not manufactured by the body.

Estrogens—These are also known as the female hormones of which there are three distinct forms: estrone, estradiol, and estriol.

Ether—A gas used as an anesthetic.

Etoposide—A plant-source class of chemotherapy also known as VePesid.

External Beam—A specific type of radiation therapy.

Ewing's sarcoma—A form of cancer involving the bones of children and adolescents.

FAM—A chemotherapy regimen of 5-fluorouracil, doxorubicin, and mitomycin C.

FAMTX—A combination of 5-FU, doxorubicin, mitomycin C methotrexate, and leucovorin.

Fatty acids—Dietary fats that are essential in maintaining a healthy metabolism.

Fentanyl—A pain medication.

Fiber—Essential elements that have no nutrient value but add to the bulking of the stool and aid in cholesterol excretion.

Fibrosis—Scar tissue that forms in response to injury or occurring in places where it doesn't normally occur.

Filgrastim—Also known as the colony-stimulating factor drug Neupogen. It is classified as a biological agent.

Flare—A term to describe common side effects of hormonal anticancer drugs.

Flow cytometry—Examines individual cells as they pass through a detector system. Measures the growth and aggressiveness of tumor cells.

Floxuridine—An antimetabolite chemotherapy agent also known as 5-FUDR.

Fludaribine—An antimetabolite class chemotherapy agent also known as FLUDARA.

Fluoxymesterol—An anticancer hormone biological agent also known as Halotestin.

Flutamide—An anticancer hormonal agent also known as Eulexin.

Folate—A vitamin in the B family of vitamins essential for healthy production of red blood cells and white blood cells and a vital nutrient in keeping genetic DNA and RNA healthy.

Folinic acid—A molecule capable of adding or removing an electron from a human cell and thus damaging the cell. Certain chemotherapy agents and radiation therapies use folinic acid to sensitize tumor cells and make them more susceptible to the therapy.

Fungicide—An agent used to kill molds and fungus. These are highly toxic to human cells and carcinogenic.

Gemcitabine—An antimetabolite chemotherapy agent also known as Gemzar.

Gemcitabine—An antimetabolite chemotherapy agent also known as Gemzar.

Glioma—A tumor that is found in the nervous system.

Glucose—Also known as blood sugar in the body.

Goserelin—Also known as Zoladex, a hormonal chemotherapeutic agent that has anticancer properties.

Granulocyte—A white blood cell that is part of the defense system of the body.

Graft versus host disease—A condition that results after bone marrow transplant the transplanted cells attack the body's cells. Also known as graft rejection.

Growth factors—These are biological active agents that stimulate the bone marrow to produce blood cells.

Growth hormone—A pituitary gland secreted hormone that stimulates growth in cells and tissues of the body.

Hematopoiesis—The formation of new red blood cells.

Hematologist—A specialist that studies and treats blood disorders including cancer.

Hematology—The study of blood and the testing of whole blood and serum. Otherwise known as a CBC, platelet count, and differential.

Hepatic—Anatomical term that relates to the liver.

Hepatobilliary System—Anatomical term to describe the liver, gallbladder, and biliary system that delivers bile to the small intestine.

Hepatoma—Also known as cancer of the liver.

Hepatotoxic—Toxicity that can potentially harm the liver and its physiological function.

Herpes—A virus family that causes health conditions like Epstein-Barr Virus (chronic fatigue), mouth sores, and genital herpes.

Hodgkin's Disease—A cancer that affects the lymph nodes, liver, and spleen.

Homeopathic medicine—A system of medicine that uses the theory "like cures like"—a small amount of a substance provides a potentially curative response in the body.

Hormone—A biochemical formed in the body that travels and delivers a message to another part of the body where it facilitates a particular function.

Hydrocodone—A drug that is used in pain management.

Hydromorphone—A drug that is used in pain management.

Hydroxyurea—An antimetabolite chemotherapy drug.

Hypercalcemia—Elevation of the mineral calcium in the blood.

Hypertension—Also known as high blood pressure.

Hyperthermia—Higher than normal body temperature.

Hypervitaminosis—A condition that results from toxic levels of certain vitamins, mainly vitamin A.

Hypocalcemia—Low blood calcium.

Hypotension—Low blood pressure.

Idarubicin—An antitumor antibiotic chemotherapeutic agent.

Ifosfamide—An alkylating chemotherapeutic agent.

Immune system—The system of the body that is involved with defense against harmful agents. It involves the thymus, lymph, spleen, and bone marrow.

Immune System Suppression—Also known as bone marrow suppression that leads to depressed immune factors necessary for defense. In addition, the result of therapy either to intentionally inhibit a specific immune function or the result of adverse reaction of therapy.

Immunoglobulin—Immune defense proteins also known as IgA, IgD, IgE, IgG and IgM. These proteins attack foreign antigens.

Infection—An organism that does not belong in a certain part of the body or that is in greater than normal levels.

Infertility—Inability to reproduce or conceive.

Insulin—A hormone that is produced by the pancreas to assist in the regulation of blood sugar.

Interferons—Biologically active substances that regulate and potentiate cell production and function.

Interleukins—Biologically active substances that regulate and potentiate function in the immune system.

Irinotecan—A plant-derived chemotherapeutic agent.

Ischemia—Reduction of blood supply to a particular organ or part of the body.

Islet Cells—Cells that are found in the pancreas that have a specific action and function.

Leucovorin—Known as the physiological active form of a B vitamin known as folic acid. It is considered a chemnotherapuetic agent and used to assist in the recovery of depleted folic acid levels that result from the use of other agents, i.e methotrexate.

Leukemia—A cancer that affects the normal production of white blood cells.

Leukopenia—A condition where there is a reduction of health white blood cells.

Leukoplakia—A precancerous condition that manifests as white patches or spots in the mouth. This condition can also be seen in immune system suppression.

Leuprolide—An anticancer hormone also known as Lupron. It is considered a biological chemotherapeutic agent.

Levamisole—A biological chemotherapeutic agent. It is also known as Ergamisol.

Live blood cell analysis—A blood test that is used as an adjunctive tool to assist in designing a more specific integrative cancer treatment plan. It is not considered a diagnostic form of testing. This test utilizes Darkfield microscopy.

Lomustine—Also known as CCNU a chemotherapeutic alkylating agent.

L-PAM—Also known as melphalan.

L-Sarcolysin—Also known as melphalan.

Lymphocyte—A white blood cell that is involved with immune defense and function.

Lymphedema—Swelling caused by fluid that accumulates in body tissue normally drained by the lymph nodes. This condition is experienced in cancers that affect lymph drainage and/or surgical procedures that remove a portion of the lymph system.

Lymphoma—A cancer that involves the lymph system and lymph glands.

Lymphorecticuloma—Another name for Hodgkin's disease, a common cancer of the lymphatic system.

MABCDP—A chemotherapeutic regime that combines methotrexate, doxorubicin, bleomycin, cyclophosphamide, dactinomycin, and cisplatin.

MRI—An imaging technique that creates a magnetic field in the body and measures the disruption of the body field. It is mainly used to define disease that affects the soft tissue of the body.

MAID—A chemotherapeutic regimen that combines mesna, doxorubicin, ifosfamide, and dacarbazine.

Malignancy—A term used to describe cancer.

Malignant effusion—Body fluid that contains active cancer cells.

Malnutrition—Inadequate nutrition to maintain normal body function.

Mechlorethamine—A chemotherapeutic alkylating agent also known as Mustargen.

Melanoma—A virulent skin cancer.

Melphalan—A chemotherapeutic alkylating agent also known as L-PAM.

Mentation—The ability to comprehend and process information.

Mercaptopurine—An antimetabolite chemotherapeutic agent also known as Purinethol.

Mesna—An antioxidant drug used to protect the urinary tract from toxicity that results from the use of alkylating chemotherapeutic agents.

Metastatic disease—Cancer spread to a site distant from the primary tumor.

Methotrexate—An antimetabolite chemotherapeutic agent also known as Folex.

Micrometastases—Tumor cells that are small free-floating cells.

Micronutrient—A nutrient that is required by the body for normal function but is only necessary in smaller amounts.

Mineral—A naturally occurring element needed for human nutrition.

Mitomycin—An antitumor antibiotic chemotherapeutic agent that is also known as Mitomycin C and Mutamycin.

Mitotane—A chemotherapeutic agent primarily used in adrenal tumors.

Mitoxanthrone—An antitumor, antibiotic chemotherapeutic agent also known as Novanthrone.

MOPP—A chemotherapeutic combination regimen of mechlorethamine, vincristine, procarbazine, and prednisone.

Morphine—A drug used in pain management.

Mucositis—Mouth sores caused by chemotherapy. This is a reversible condition.

Multiple interaction pathways—Both conventional and nonconventional treatments working together in multiple cancers.

Mutation—Cancer cells that have changed in character and expression genetically.

M-VAC—A chemotherapeutic combination therapy that include the drugs methotrexate, vinblastine, doxorubicin and cisplatin.

MVP—A chemotherapeutic combination therapy that include the drugs mitomycin, vinblastine, doxorubicin and cisplatin.

Myeloma—A cancer composed of cells normally found in the bone marrow.

Myelosuppression—Bone marrow doesn't produce the cell lines needed to keep the blood healthy and strong. Chemotherapeutic agents, radiation therapy, and certain cancer types can cause this to occur.

Myoclonus—Spasm or twitching of muscle.

Myopathy—Disease of the skeletal muscle.

Naturopathy—A system of medicine that integrates herbal, nutritional, metabolic, and immune modulating therapies, observing the six guiding principles of naturopathic medicine, starting with "first do no harm."

Nephritis—Inflammation of the kidney.

Neuroendocrine system—The nervous system combined with the body's glandular system to control the secretion of hormones.

Neuropathy—Diseases that affect the nerves.

Neurotoxicity—Poisonous to the nervous system.

Neutropenia—Low levels of certain white blood cells known as neutrophils.

Nitrosurea—An alkylating chemotherapeutic agent.

Nodes negative—Cancer spread is not detected in the lymph nodes.

Non-Hodgkin's Lymphoma—Lymphoma that does not have the characteristic Reed-Sternberg cells found in Hodgkin's disease.

Non-ionizing radiation—Magnetic fields that surround power lines and any other electrical conduction system.

Nutrient—An essential substance that the body needs for nourishment to maintain health.

Nutrition—The processes involved in dietary intake that maintain healthy body function.

Obesity—Excess weight that can interfere with healthy body function.

Octeotride—A biological chemotherapeutic agent.

Oncologist—A specialist in cancer medicine.

Osteosarcoma—A cancer that affects immature bone tissue.

Osteopath—A physician trained as a medical practitioner with special emphasis on spinal manipulation.

Ovary—An anatomical term to describe a female gland responsible for reproduction.

Oxycodone—A pain management drug.

Ozone—A three-molecule oxygen as compared to the readily occurring two-molecule oxygen. Ozone therapy utilizes the three-molecule oxygen. Higher amounts of ozone is known to pollute the atmosphere. Ozone's harmful effects are ambiguous and highly controversial.

Paclitaxel—A plant-derived chemotherapeutic agent also known as Taxol.

Pancreas—An anatomical term to describe a vital organ of the body that helps to regulate many physiological functions of the body.

Papillary carcinoma—A slow-growing thyroid cancer.

Parasympathetic nervous system—The rest, relax, repose portion of the nervous system.

PE—A chemotherapy combination that includes cisplatin and etoposide.

PEB—A chemotherapy combination that includes cisplatin, etoposide, and bleomycin.

Pentostatin—Also known as NIPENT, which is a antimetabolite chemotherapeutic agent.

Pericarditis—Inflammation of the sac surrounding the heart.

Peripheral neuropathy—Numbness of the hands and feet that can occur in specific health conditions including cancer and adverse effects of conventional therapies used in cancer treatment.

Peripheral stem cell transplantation—A specific form of bone marrow transplant that replaces immature cells rather than marrow cells.

Peritoneum—An anatomical term to describe the membrane surrounding the inside of the abdomen and pelvis.

Pesticide—Chemicals linked to causing some forms of cancer and used to kill insects.

PET scan—A specific imaging method that uses an isotope tracer and monitors gamma rays emitted to enhance a specific field of view within the body.

Platelet—Cells formed within the bone marrow responsible for the clotting of blood.

Pleura—An anatomical term used to describe the membrane that surrounds the lung.

Pleural effusion—Fluid accumulation inside the pleura of the lung.

Plicamycin—An antitumor antibiotic chemotherapeutic agent also known as Mithracin.

Pneumonia—Inflammation of the lungs.

Positive lymph node—Indicates that cancer cells are found within the lymph node and indicates spread from the primary site.

Prednisone—A drug in the steroid category.

Pressor—Foods that can augment the efficacy of drugs that inhibit the monoamine oxidase pathways.

Procarbazine—An alkylating chemotherapeutic agent also known as Matulane and MIH.

ProMACW-CytaBOM—A combination chemotherapeutic regimen.

Prostaglandin—Biochemical agents found in the body that are involved with inflammation response, blood vessel constriction and dilation, reduced platelet aggregation, and histamine response.

Prostate gland—An anatomical term that describes a gland found in males. This gland is responsible for secreting and delivery of seminal fluid that carries sperm. A common site for cancer in males.

Proteins—Complex compounds in the body and in foods necessary to serve as enzymes, hormones, immunoglobulins (immune defense proteins), and other functions.

Pruritis—Itching associated with drug reaction or a specific health condition including cancer.

Pulmonary—Pertaining to the lung.

Pulmonary edema—Fluid in the lungs.

Radiation—A form of high-energy particles used in cancer treatment to destroy tumor cells.

Radiation oncologist—A specialist of oncology who provides radiation therapy.

Radon—A colorless active gas naturally occurring in nature used in radiation therapy.

Raynaud's Phenomenon—Intermittent attacks of reduced blood flow to the hand and feet resulting in cold limbs and numbness. Heat usually relieves this condition.

RDA—Recommended daily allowance of nutrients, vitamins, and minerals. This recommendation by no means addresses biochemical individuality.

Renal—An anatomical term for kidney.

Rescues—Treatments designed to undo toxicity of a prior treatment.

Retina—The lining of the back of the eye where image is focused and the signal transmitted to the brain.

Retinoic Acid—A chemotherapeutic agent similar to vitamin A.

Retinoid—A substance that has chemical activity similar to vitamin A.

Salivary gland—Glands that surround the mouth producing saliva, which is responsible for the lubrication and pre-digestion of food.

Sarcoma—Tumors that have their origins from connective tissue, muscle, bone, and skin.

Sargramostim—A biological chemotherapeutic agent also known as Leukine and Prokine.

Schwann cells—Cells that are the source of myelin, which is a protein responsible for the development of the protective insulator around nerve cells and that keeps them from short-circuiting.

Seizure—An event that involves the nervous system where there is a loss of consciousness, loss of muscle control, convulsion, and/or other malfunction.

Sentinel node biopsy—A procedure in which one or a few lymph nodes are removed for diagnosis.

Sepsis—A term to describe an infection of the blood.

SMAC—A term that describes blood test that are specific to blood chemistries.

Sputum—A mucus matter that is spit out through the mouth from the lungs or can also result from chronic esophageal irritation (gastric reflux).

Staging—Tumor classification with respect to how far they have progressed and the potential to responding to treatment.

Stem cell—A precursor cell in the bone marrow responsible for facilitating and producing mature cell lines found in the blood.

Steroid—A hormone agent found in nature and the human body.

Streptozocin—An alkylating chemotherapeutic agent.

Sympathetic nervous system—The part of the nervous system responsible for the fight or flight response. This is the system that responds to immediate crisis of the body.

Tamoxifen—An antihormonal chemotherapeutic agent with specific antiestrogenic properties.

Taxol—See paclitaxel.

Temozolide—An alkylating chemotherapeutic agent.

Teniposide—A plant-derived chemotherapeutic agent also known as Vumon.

Therapeutic window—Also known as the therapeutic index. The range of dosage that produces that greatest therapeutic results. The lower limits are the minimal dose that has the desired therapeutic effects. The maximum dose is beyond which side effects are undesirable.

Thioguanine—An antimetabolite chemotherapeutic agent also known as 6-TG.

Thiotepa—An alkylating chemotherapeutic agent.

Thorax—An anatomical term describing the neck, abdomen, and chest.

Thrombocytopenia—Decreased number of platelets in the blood.

Thyroid—A gland in the neck that regulates metabolic rate in the body and calcium uptake in the bone.

TNM—A classification system used for the staging of cancer. More specifically, tumor size and character, lymph node involvement, and distant metastasis.

Total Parenteral Nutrition (TPN)—A source of nutrition administered intravenously.

Transurethral resection—A surgical procedure where the surgeon enters through the urethra.

Treatment response—Data describing cases where cancer regressed in response to a specific treatment.

Tumor markers—Substances in blood that indicate malignant growth.

Ultrasound—An imaging technique that uses sound to provide a picture of a specific area of the body.

Urinalysis—The examination of the urine for a variety of chemicals, proteins, and other contents for diagnostic evaluation.

Urinary tract—The organs and pathways of the body that carry urine. The kidneys, bladder, and urethra are all involved in this process.

Uterus—A hollow, pear-shaped organ found in females where the fertilized egg normally implants and develops.

VAB-6—A combination chemotherapeutic regimen that includes vinblastine, cyclophosphamide, dactinomycin, bleomycin, and cisplatin.

VACD—A combination chemotherapeutic regimen that includes vincristine, doxorubicin, cyclophosphamide, and dactinomycin.

Vanderbuilt Regimen—A combination of chemotherapeutic agents.

VATH—A combination of chemotherapeutic agents including vinblastine, doxorubicin, thiotepa, and fluoxymesterone.

VBMCP—A combination of chemotheapeutic agents—See appendix.

Vinblastine—A plant-derived chemotherapeutic agent also known as Velban and Velsar.

Vincristine—A plant-derived chemotherapeutic agent also known as Oncovin.

Vinorelbine—A plant-derived chemotherapeutic agent also known as Navelbine.

Vitamin—A substance found in food necessary for the healthy function of the body. Vitamins are derived from the diet and, when taken as a nonfood source, require food to be metabolically used in the body.

Whipple procedure—A surgical procedure used in pancreatic cancer that involves the removal of the lower part of the stomach, a section of the small intestine, and part of the pancreas.

X-ray—Imaging using an ionizing form of radiation to highlight specific areas of the body. X-ray cannot penetrate all parts of the body and has its limitations. X-ray is one of the oldest imaging procedures in existence in modern medicine.

For more information contact:

Health&Wellness Institute®, Inc.
5603 - 230th Street S.W.
Mountlake Terrace, WA 98043
www.ehealthandhealing.com

Index

Symbols

2-Deoxycoformycin 315
5-Fluorouracil 315
5-FUDR 315
6-MP 315
6-TG. 315

A

abdominal pain 206
ablative oophorectomy 315
ABVD 92, 315
acemannan 205
acetaminophen 218, 222
acid-base balance 105
acid/alkaline diets 197
acidophilus 188
acupuncture 50, 52, 244, 246, 315
adaptogen 315
adenopathy 316
adrenal cortical carcinoma 316
adrenal support formula 200
Adriamycin 139, 282, 299, 316, 323
aflatoxin 316

I

M

Q

R

About the Author

Dr. John A. Catanzaro, president and founder of the Health&Wellness Institute®, is a naturopathic physician who received his education and training at Bastyr University, America's leading university in alternative medicine. He has a staff of three physicians at Health&Wellness Institute® in Mountlake Terrace, Washington. Dr. Catanzaro began Health &Wellness with the model of personalized health care, and his vision is to expand this new model and focus to restore the empathy in medical care. Health&Wellness's focus is on the whole person, which includes the physical body, soul, and spirit. Quality care with compassion and putting the soul back in medicine is the mission statement of Health&Wellness Institute®.

Another arm is to provide new physicians, who are just graduating, with on-the-job clinical experience, which builds confidence and inspiration to move forward and practice the medicine that comes from within their soul. He is committed to training new physicians in the field of integrative medicine and providing quality health care in the process. He currently serves as vice chair of the Naturopathic Advisory Committee for Washington State Health Care Quality Assurance Board. He is also a consultant on matters of health care quality in the corporate and public sector. Dr. Catanzaro is also an ordained minister with expertise in emotional and spiritual matters, which effect total health. He strongly believes in the miracle and power of healing ordained by God and has seen many miracles take place in the individual life experiences of patients he has had the privilege to treat.

Dr. Catanzaro, from a young boy, wanted to be a doctor and is now doing what he envisioned. He is married to Anna, with whom he has celebrated their twenty-fifth anniversary, and they have five children, two boys and three girls. The oldest of their children, both sons, are twenty-four and the youngest is eight. His family is his priority and he models this no matter how challenging his schedule may be. For it is the team effort of his family members that contributes to the success of Dr. Catanzaro's endeavors. Dr. Catanzaro's hobbies include music (drum and keyboard), airplanes, and baseball. He is currently completing another book entitled *Jesus Still Heals the Sick,* which is scheduled to be published next year. The focus of this work is the soul and spirit of healing from a Christian perspective.

Upcoming books By Dr. John A. Catanzaro:

Jesus Still Heals the Sick

Mapping our Spiritual Genes

Minibooks (Minibooks are available from Health&Wellness Institute®):

* *The Journey Toward Healing*

* *Experiencing Health*

[1] Committee on Diet, Nutrition and Cancer. Assembly of Life Sciences, National Research Council. *Diet, Nutrition and Cancer.* Washington, DC: National Academy Press, 1982.

[2] Weinstein, A.L., et al. "Breast Cancer Risk and Oral Contraceptive Use: Results from a Large Case-Control Study." *Epidemiology* 2:5 (September 1991): 353–358.

To order additional copies of

CANCER

AN INTEGRATIVE
APPROACH

Have your credit card ready and call

Toll free: (877) 421-READ (7323)

or send $19.95* each plus $5.95 S&H** to

**WinePress Publishing
PO Box 428
Enumclaw, WA 98022**

or order online at: www.winepressbooks.com

*Washington residents, add 8.4% sales tax
**add $1.50 S&H for each additional book ordered